(100)

Nuclear Ophthalmology

Wiley Series in Diagnostic and Therapeutic Radiology

Luther W. Brady, M.D., Editor
Professor and Chairman, Department of Therapeutic Radiology and Nuclear Medicine, Hahnemann Medical College and Hospital, Philadelphia, Pennsylvania

TUMORS OF THE NERVOUS SYSTEM
   Edited by H. Gunter Seydel, M.D., M.S.

CANCER OF THE LUNG
   By H. Gunter Seydel, M.D., M.S.
   Arnold Chait, M.D.
   John T. Gmelich, M.D.

CLINICAL APPLICAITONS OF THE ELECTRON BEAM
   Edited by Norah duV. Tapley, M.D.

NUCLEAR OPHTHALMOLOGY
   Edited by Millard N. Croll, M.D.
   Luther W. Brady, M.D.
   Paul Carmichael, M.D.
   Robert J. Wallner, D.O.

HIGH-ENERGY PHOTONS AND ELECTRONS:
Clinical Applications in Cancer Management
   Edited by Simon Kramer, M.D.
   Nagalingam Suntharalingam, Ph.D.
   George F. Zinninger, M.D.

Nuclear Ophthalmology

Edited by

Millard N. Croll, M.D.
Luther W. Brady, M.D.
Paul Carmichael, M.D.
Robert J. Wallner, D.O.

A WILEY MEDICAL PUBLICATION

JOHN WILEY & SONS
New York / London / Sydney / Toronto

Copyright © 1976 by John Wiley & Sons, Inc.

All rights reserved. Published simultaneously in Canada.

No part of this book may be reproduced by any means,
nor transmitted, nor translated into a machine language
without the written permission of the publisher.

Library of Congress Cataloging in Publication Data:

Main entry under title:

Nuclear ophthalmology.

   (Wiley series in diagnostic and therapeutic radiology)
(A Wiley Medical publication)
   Includes bibliographical references.
   1. Radioisotopes in ophthalmology. 2. Eye—Diseases
and defects—Diagnosis. 3. Eye—Tumors—Diagnosis.
I. Croll, Millard N.

RE79.R33N8   617.7'1   76-7088
ISBN 0-471-01388-9

Printed in the United States of America

10 9 8 7 6 5 4 3 2 1

Contributors

William Annesley, M.D., Clinical Professor of Ophthalmology, Thomas Jefferson University; Chief, Retina Service, Wills Eye Hospital, Philadelphia, Pennsylvania

Harold L. Atkins, M.D., Senior Scientist, Medical Department, Brookhaven National Laboratory, Upton, Long Island, New York

Paul Blanquet, M.D., Director, de L'Unite de Recherches, Inserm, Bordeaux, France

D. Blanc, M.D., L'Unite de Recherches, Inserm, Bordeaux, France

Luther W. Brady, M.D., Professor and Chairman, Department of Radiation Therapy and Nuclear Medicine, Hahnemann Medical College, Philadelphia, Pennsylvania

Joseph Bronzino, Ph.D., Clinical Consultant, Biological Engineering, University of Connecticut Health Center, Farmington, Connecticut

Gerald A. Bruno, Ph.D., Director, Diagnostic Research and Development Department, The Squibb Institute for Medical Research, New Brunswick, New Jersey

Paul L. Carmichael, M.D., Clinical Associate Professor, Department of Radiation Therapy and Nuclear Medicine, Hahnemann Medical College; Assistant Surgeon, Retina Service, Wills Eye Hospital, Philadelphia, Pennsylvania

Arthur C. Chandler, M.D., Associate Professor of Ophthalmology, Associate in Anatomy, Department of Ophthalmology, Duke University Medical Center, Durham, North Carolina

Millard N. Croll, M.D., Professor of Radiation Therapy and Nuclear Medicine, Director, Nuclear Medicine, Hahnemann Medical College, Philadelphia, Pennsylvania

Donald P. D'Amato, Ph.D., Assistant Professor of Ophthalmology, Division of Ophthalmology, University of Connecticut Health Center, Farmington, Connecticut

Gehangir Durrani, M.D., Assistant Professor of Ophthalmology, Division of Ophthalmology, University of Connecticut Health Center; Chief of Ophthalmology, Veterans Hospital, Farmington, Connecticut

Jay L. Federman, M.D., Senior Assistant Surgeon, Wills Eye Hospital; Assistant Professor of Ophthalmology, Thomas Jefferson University, Philadelphia, Pennsylvania

Joseph C. Flanagan, M.D., Senior Assistant Surgeon, Oculoplastic Service, Wills Eye Hospital; Clinical Associate Professor, Thomas Jefferson University, Philadelphia, Pennsylvania

Richard Goldberg, M.D., Associate Surgeon, Retina Service, Wills Eye Hospital; Clinical Associate Professor of Ophthalmology, Thomas Jefferson University, Philadelphia, Pennsylvania

Jack K. Goodrich, Ph.D., Professor of Radiology, Director, Division of Nuclear Medicine, Department of Radiology, Duke University Medical Center, Durham, North Carolina

Arthur S. Grove, M.D., Instructor in Ophthalmology, Harvard Medical School, Boston, Massachusetts

Robert B. Grove, M.D., Director of Nuclear Medicine, Ireland Army Hospital, Fort Knox, Kentucky

C. Craig Harris, M.S., Associate Professor of Radiology, Division of Nuclear Medicine, Department of Radiology, Duke University Medical Center, Durham, North Carolina

Ned D. Heindel, Ph.D., Professor of Chemistry, Lehigh University; Associate Professor, Department of Radiation Therapy and Nuclear Medicine, Hahnemann Medical College, Philadelphia, Pennsylvania

Ernest E. Howerton, Jr., M.D., Resident in Ophthalmology, Department of Ophthalmology, University of Texas Medical School, Houston, Texas

William Jarrett II, M.D., Clinical Associate Professor of Ophthalmology, Medical School of Georgia, Augusta, Georgia

Jane K. Keiser, R.T., Senior Nuclear Medicine Technologist, Division of Nuclear Medicine, Department of Radiology, Duke University Medical Center, Durham, North Carolina

Richard M. Lambrecht, Ph.D., Chemist, Brookhaven National Laboratory, Upton, Long Island, New York

Brian C. Leonard, M.D., FRCS (C), Assistant Professor of Ophthalmology, University of Ottawa, Ottawa, Canada

M. J. LeRebeller, M.D., Service d'Ophthalmologie, Hopital Saint-Andre, Bordeaux, France

P. Robb McDonald, M.D., Consultant, Retina Service, Wills Eye Hospital; Professor of Ophthalmology, Thomas Jefferson University, Philadelphia, Pennsylvania

Charles Miller, M.D., Clinical Associate of Theoretical Physics, Department of Ophthalmology, University of Connecticut Health Center, Farmington, Connecticut

James F. O'Rourke, M.D., Professor and Chairman, Department of Ophthalmology, University of Connecticut Health Center, Farmington, Connecticut

Samuel Packer, M.D., Clinical Instructor, Department of Ophthalmology, Cornell University School of Medicine, Manhattan, New York

W. Leslie Rogers, Ph.D., Assistant Professor of Internal Medicine, Division of Nuclear Medicine, University of Michigan Medical Center, Ann Arbor, Michigan

Richard S. Ruiz, M.D., Clinical Professor of Ophthalmology, University of Texas Medical School, Houston, Texas

Lov Sarin, M.D., Associate Surgeon, Retina Service, Wills Eye Hospital; Clinical Professor of Ophthalmology, Thomas Jefferson University, Philadelphia, Pennsylvania

N. Safi, M.D., Hopital Pellegrin, Service des Istotopes, Place Amelie Raba-Leon, Bordeaux, France

Ijaz Shafi, M.D., Assistant Professor of Ophthalmology, University of Connecticut Health Center, Division of Ophthalmology, Farmington, Connecticut

Jerry Shields, M.D., Senior Assistant Surgeon, Retina Service, Wills Eye Hospital, Philadelphia, Pennsylvania

James Sisson, M.D., Professor of Internal Medicine, Section of Nuclear Medicine, University of Michigan Medical Center, Ann Arbor, Michigan

E. Thoreson, M.D., Hopital Pellegrin, Service des Isotopes, Place Amelie Raba-Leon, Bordeaux, France

Alfred P. Wolf, Ph.D., Senior Scientist of Chemistry, Brookhaven National Laboratory, Upton, Long Island, New York

Michael A. Wainstock, M.D., Clinical Assistant Professor in Ophthalmology, Director of Ultrasonic Laboratory, University of Michigan Medical Center, Ann Arbor, Michigan

Robert J. Wallner, D.O., Assistant Professor of Radiation Therapy and Nuclear Medicine, Hahnemann Medical College, Philadelphia, Pennsylvania

John Weiter, M.D., Research Associate, Naval Medical Center, Bethesda, Maryland

Series Preface

The past five years have produced an explosion in the knowledge, techniques, and clinical application of radiology in all of its specialties. New techniques in diagnostic radiology have contributed to a quality of medical care for the patient unparalleled in the United States. Among these techniques are the development and applications in ultrasound, the development and implementation of computed tomography, and many exploratory studies using holographic techniques. The advances in nuclear medicine have allowed for a wider diversity of application of these techniques in clinical medicine and have involved not only major new developments in instrumentation, but also development of newer radiopharmaceuticals.

Advances in radiation therapy have significantly improved the cure rates for cancer. Radiation techniques in the treatment of cancer are now utilized in more than 50% of the patients with the established diagnosis of cancer.

It is the purpose of this series of monographs to bring together the various aspects of radiology and all its specialties so that the physician by continuance of his education and rigid self-discipline may maintain high standards of professional knowledge.

LUTHER W. BRADY, M.D.

Preface

Since the introduction of radioactive phosphorus in the treatment of a patient with polycythemia vera in 1937, the growth in the utilization of radioactive nuclides for diagnosis and treatment in human diseases has been dramatic. Almost all disciplines in medicine have made diagnostic use of radionuclides, some to a greater extent than others. The application of nuclear medical techniques to ophthalmology has been gradual and for the most part, unreported. Until recently, most activity in this area was limited to radiophosphorus localization of eye tumors. The availability of multiple short-lived nuclides along with the development of sophisticated detection instrumentation has permitted extensive application of these techniques to diseases of the eye.

The latest developments in static and dynamic radionuclide techniques were presented at a unique symposium, Nuclear Ophthalmology, held at the Hahnemann Medical College and Hospital on March 7-8, 1975 and jointly sponsored by the Department of Radiation Therapy and Nuclear Medicine of Hahnemann Medical College and the Retina Service of the Wills Eye Hospital. The purpose of the symposium was to bring together prominent investigators in both nuclear medicine and ophthalmology to share in the information derived from new radionuclide techniques applied to the problems of ophthalmology. It is the editors' firm belief that this was accomplished.

A special debt of gratitude is due to the Medotopes® Division of E. R. Squibb and Sons for its financial support of the symposium.

The editors are grateful to the contributors for their willingness to undertake the task of committing their comments to a written text and their patience with our persistent stimuli for completion of their manuscript. We are appreciative of the help given by the publishers in the preparation of the volume, and we are grateful as well as to Mr. Carl Karsch, Ms. Jane Cappiello, Mrs. Gloria Sword (R.T.NMT), and Ms. Diane Regan (R.T.NMT) for their able and patient editorial and technical assistance.

Our sincere appreciation is extended to Dr. Thomas Duane, Ophthalmologist-in-Chief, Wills Eye Hospital and Professor of Ophthalmology, Thomas Jefferson University, and to Dr. William Annesley, Chief of the Retina Service, Wills Eye Hospital and Clinical Professor of Ophthalmology, Thomas Jefferson University for their support of the symposium.

MILLARD N. CROLL
LUTHER W. BRADY
PAUL CARMICHAEL
ROBERT J. WALLNER

Philadelphia, Pennsylvania
March 1976

Contents

Nuclear Ophthalmology

Introduction

Paul L. Carmichael, M.D.
Department of Radiation Therapy
and Nuclear Medicine,
Hahnemann Medical College;
Associate Surgeon, Retina Service,
Wills Eye Hospital,
Philadelphia, Pennsylvania

Millard N. Croll, M.D.
Professor of Radiation Therapy
and Nuclear Medicine,
Hahnemann Medical College,
Philadelphia, Pennsylvania

The field of nuclear medicine has expanded remarkably in the past 15 years. Technological and pharmaceutical innovations have made it possible to explore dynamic physiological functions previously unknown to clinicians and research investigators. Although most of the specialties in medicine have benefited greatly from the knowledge garnered from a multiplicity of organ and topographical studies, the specialty of ophthalmology has only recently derived clinical benefit from the use of routine radionuclide studies.

Although Kinsey and co-workers[1] utilized radioisotopes in their investigations of aqueous humor dynamics and Thomas[2] introduced the use of radioactive phosphorous as a clinical test for the diagnosis of uveal melanomas, the contributions made by nuclear medicine to clinical ophthalmology continued to remain somewhat sparse until the introduction of newer radiopharmaceuticals and detectors. The problem has been the anatomical size of the globe (23.5 mm) and orbit (35 × 40 × 40 mm). The resolution of radioactive emissions from so small an area tends to obscure information that would be useful to the ophthalmologist. Because of the limitation imposed by gamma emitters, the beta emitter ^{32}P continued to be used for many years as a useful tool for the detection of uveal melanomas.[3-6] However, limitations imposed by the necessity for invasive surgical techniques in order to insure accurate detection[7, 8] of tumors led to further study of the use of newer, short-lived radiopharmaceuticals which could lead to imaging of tumors or the use of noninvasive counting techniques with specially designed detectors.[9, 10]

Geiger-Mueller detectors for beta radiation have been in use for many years in the clinical investigation of uveal melanomas.[11] Recently, a solid-state lithium drifted silicon detector has been introduced which is also a serviceable clinical instrument. An excellent review of the physical peculiarities of these detectors has been presented by La Rose.[12] Rectilinear scanners and gamma cameras are in use for studying the orbits and the surrounding areas. Special scintillation probes have been designed for studies with ^{125}I chloroquine[1] and for ^{99m}Tc studies of the lacrimal apparatus.[13] It is possible that in the near future, the combination of a short-lived radionuclide and a semiconductor camera detector may be the best system for imaging techniques of the globe and its contents.

TABLE 1

Radionuclide	IV Dose	Half-Life	Radiation	MeV	Critical Organ	Dose to Critical Organ	Total Body Dose
^{32}P Sodium phosphate	500–750 µCi	14.3 days	β^-	1.72	Blood Bone marrow	14.2 rads	5.24 rad
^{197}Hg Chlormerodrin	750 µCi	2.7 days	γ	0.77	Kidney	13 rads	0.08 rad
^{131}I albumin (or DIF)	375 µCi	8.0 days	β^- γ	0.608 0.364	Blood	2 rads	0.04 rad
^{203}Hg Chlormerodrin	750 µCi	47.9 days	β^- γ	0.214 0.280	Kidney	165 rads	0.18 rad
^{99m}Technetium pertechnetate	15 mCi	6.0 hours	γ	0.140	Large bowel	1–3 rads	0.18 rad
^{125}I chloroquine	2–4 mCi oral	60.0 days	γ	0.213	Eye	46 rads	
^{67}Gallium citrate	3 mCi	78.0 hours	γ	0.296	Bone Liver	2.0 rads 1.8 rads	0.31 rad

Table 1 lists the more commonly used radionuclides in ophthalmology and their characteristics. It can be seen that the shorter lived radionuclides lend themselves more readily to imaging procedures, especially those of the orbital and adnexal areas.[14, 15, 16] Investigators will continue to seek out and utilize newer, short-lived radionuclides as they become available. Because of the development of integrative techniques utilizing detector-radiopharmaceutical relationships with specialized viewing methods,[17] the orbital areas and structures such as the lacrimal apparatus have been studied successfully with radionuclides.

Studies of anatomical areas of specific interest to the ophthalmologist have been advanced by adaptation of flow study techniques already in use by nuclear medicine laboratories.[18, 19] Probably the most advanced detection techniques are those presented by O'Rourke and D'Amato in this volume. These promise to further clarify the physiology of ocular microcirculation and may be found useful for many other research projects in ocular physiology.

The future of ophthalmic nuclear medicine appears to be secure. Continued expansion into fields allied with clinical nuclear medicine and investigative research is a certainty. It will be the field most likely to lead nuclear medicine into the study of microphysiological techniques because of the necessity for their use in an organ so small and complex as the human eye. The studies of the many distinguished clinicians and investigators who have contributed to this unique volume have already secured the basis for the further advancement of nuclear ophthalmology.

REFERENCES

1. Baraney, E., and Kinsey, V., The Rate of Flow of Aqueous Humor; Rate of Disappearance of Para-amino Hippuric Acid, Radioactive Rayopake, and Radioactive Diodrast from the Aqueous Humor of Rabbits. *Am. J. Ophthalmol.* **32**:177 (1949).

2. Thomas, C. I., Krohmer, J. S., and Storaasli, J. P.: Detection of Intraocular Tumors with Radioactive Phosphorus. *A.M.A. Arch. Ophthalmol.* **47**:276–286 (1952).

3. Bethman, J. W., and Fellows, V.: Radioactive Phosphorous as a Diagnostic Aid in Ophthalmology. *Arch. Ophthalmol.* **51**:171 (1954).

4. Terner, I. S., Leopold, I. H., and Eisenberg, I. J.: The Radioactive Phosphorous Uptake Test in Ophthalmology. *Arch. Ophthalmol.* **55**:52 (1956).

5. Carmichael, P. L., and Leopold, I. H.: Radioactive Phosphorous Test in Ophthalmology. *Am. J. Ophthalmol.* **49**:484, (1960).

6. Leopold, I. H., Keates, E. V., and Charkes, I. D.: Role of Isotope in Diagnosis of Intraocular Neoplasms. *Trans. Am. Ophthalmol. Soc.* **62**:89 (1964).

7. Hagler, W. S., Jarrett, W. H., and Humphrey, W. T.: The Radioactive Phosphorous Uptake Test in Diagnosis of Uveal Melanoma. *Arch. Ophthalmol.* **83**:548 (1970).

8. Carmichael, P. L., Holst, G. C., Federman, J. L., and Shields, J. A.: The Present Status of the ^{32}P Test in Ophthalmology. In Croll, M. N., Brady, L. W., Honda, T., and Wallner, R. J., Eds., *New Techniques in Tumor Localization and Radioimmunoassay.* John Wiley, New York, (1974).

9. Beierwaltes, W. H., Lieberman, M., Varma, V. M., and Counsell, R. E., Visualizing Human Malignant Melanoma and Metastases. Use of Chloroquine Analog Tagged with Iodine 125. *J.A.M.A.* **206**:97 (1968).

10. Knoll, G. F., Lieberm, L. M., Nishijama, H., and Beierwaltes, W. H.: A Gamma Ray Probe for the Detection of Ocular Melanomas. *IEEE Trans. Nucl. Sci.* **NS-19**:76–80 (February 1972).

11. Thomas, C. I., Krohmer, J. S., and Storaasli, J. P.: Geiger Counter Probe for Diagnosis and Localization of Posterior Intraocular Tumors. *A.M.A. Arch. Ophthalmol.* **52**:413–414 (1954).

12. La Rose, J. H.: Semiconductor Detectors for Eye Tumor Diagnosis. In Hoffer, P. B., Beck, R. N., and

Gottschalk, A., Eds., The Role of Semiconductor Detectors in the Future of Nuclear Medicine. The Society of Nuclear Medicine, New York, (1971), pp. 190–205.

13. Rossomondo, R. M., Carlton, W. H., and Trueblood, J. H.: A New Method of Evaluating Lacrimal Drainage. *Arch. Ophthamol.* **88**(5):523–525 (November 1972).

14. Trokel, S. L., Schlesinger, E. B., and Beaton, H.: Diagnosis of Orbital Tumors by Gamma Ray Orbitography. *Am. J. Ophthalmol.* **74**:675–679 (1972).

15. Grove, A. S., and Kotner, L. M.: Orbital Scanning With Multiple Radionuclides. *Arch. Ophthalmol.* **89**:301–305 (1973).

16. Grove, A. S., and Kotner, L. M.: Radionuclide Arteriography in Ophthalmology. *Arch. Ophthalmol.* **89**:13–17 (1973).

17. Wilson, E. B., and Griggs, R. C., Study of Orbital Region Using En Face View. *Radiology* 92(3):576–580 (1969).

18. Grief, R. J., Wise, G., and Marty, R.: Detection of Carotid Artery Obstruction by Intravenous Radionuclide Angiography. *Radiology* 311–316 (1970).

19. Mongeau, B.: Cerebral Blood Flow with the Multiple-Crystal Camera. In Croll, M. N., Brady, L. W., Tatem, H. R., and Honda, T., Eds., *Clinical Dynamic Function Studies with Radionuclides.* Appleton-Century-Crofts, New York, (1972), p. 151.

Physical
Fundamentals

Nuclear Medical Instrumentation

C. Craig Harris, M.S.
Associate Professor of Radiology,
Division of Nuclear Medicine,
Department of Radiology,
Duke University Medical Center,
Durham, North Carolina

The term "nuclear medical instrumentation" is used to describe those systems whose purpose is the detection of nuclear radiations (either *in vivo* with an external detector or *in vitro*), processing of the resulting electrical events, and presenting some sort of display for interpretation (image or numerical data). These systems range from the simplest—which detect radiation and present a meter indication of the intensity—to the most elaborate—those that make pictures, or images, of *in vivo* distributions of radioactivity. These hardware items are, in effect, the "tools of the trade" of nuclear medicine methodology, and some understanding of their properties is useful in any application of that methodology.

The "tools of the trade" of nuclear medicine (and of nuclear ophthalmology) have a definite, but not prohibitive, complexity. To the unitiated, their complicated natures seem even more so because of the unfamiliar language, which is colloquial, jargon, and often obscurely related to familiar uses of some of the same words. While the primary purpose of this presentation is to acquaint the reader with some basic considerations of nuclear medicine instrumentation, an emphasis will be placed on making the language of this instrumentation more familiar.

We begin, therefore, with a glossary of terms for significant items, followed by a description of specific radiation detection systems. In the glossary, certain terms that have broad or multiple meanings will be defined in the context best suited to basic considerations of radiation detection and radionuclide imaging systems. Italicization of a word indicates that it is explained further on in the glossary. Since this is a glossary, rather than a dictionary, the items are presented in order of need rather than alphabetically.

GLOSSARY

Electron.   A basic entity in atomic structure; can be considered a basic unit of negative (−) electrical charge. An electron has real mass and can be treated as a particle that has kinetic energy. Electrons normally reside in atoms by maintaining stable but dynamic energy relationships with the heavy, positively charged nucleus of the atom. The electron population in a single atom occupies specific energy levels; the electron populations of a group of closely packed atoms occupy specific bands of energy levels.

Proton.   A fundamental building block of the nuclei of atoms of matter. It is about 1840 times as heavy as an electron and possesses one unit of charge opposite (+) to that of an electron. The number of protons in a nucleus determines the chemical identity (element) of that nucleus.

Neutron.   The particle that, together with protons, forms the nuclei of atoms. A stable nucleus can possess only certain numbers and arrangements of neutrons to match its number of protons. Any departure from these numbers and arrangements results in an unstable, or "radioactive," nucleus.

Isotope.   The identification used to denote a particular variation of a chemical element, with the same proton number as all variations of that element but with a different number of neutrons. The "identification number" is the mass number, the sum of protons and neutrons in the nucleus of an atom of the element. For example, iodine-125, iodine-127, and iodine-131 are isotopes of iodine.

Radioisotope. The term used to denote isotopes that are radioactive, or unstable, and will sooner or later release their excess energy. For example, since iodine-127 is *not* radioactive, iodine-125 and iodine-131 are both radioisotopes of iodine.

Nuclide. The term used to encompass all the isotopes of all the elements. Each specific type of nucleus with any given proton number and any given neutron number is a nuclide or a member of a radionuclidic species.

Radionuclide. Any radioactive nuclide is called a "radionuclide" for short. For example, phosphorus-32, iodine-125, iodine-131, and technetium-99m are all radionuclides.

Photon. A "package" of energy that moves at the speed of light and is all energy. Gamma radiation, x-radiation, ultraviolet light, and visible light consist of photons. Photons have both electric and magnetic properties.

Gamma Ray. A photon, ejected from the unstable nucleus of an atom, specifically from a radionuclide. Often described as "penetrating electromagnetic radiation." A deexcitation radiation, its energy is that lost by the nucleus in the energy transition.

Characteristic X-rays. Electromagnetic radiations (photons) resulting from rearrangement of the electrons in an atom. They are indistinguishable from gamma rays of the same energy, and in some instances constitute the useful photon radiations from radionuclides.

Beta Particle. An electron ejected from the unstable nucleus of an atom. Energies range from zero to over 3 *MeV*. From a single radionuclidic species, energies range from zero to the energy lost by the nucleus in the energy transition that produced the beta particle.

Ionization. The removal of one or more electrons from an atom by external application of energy in the form of radiation (electrons and photons, chiefly). The residuum is a *positive ion.*

Positive Ion. That which remains when one or more electrons are removed from a normal atom. Carries one unit of positive charge for each electron removed.

Ionizing Radiation. Those forms of radiant energy having the ability and sufficient energy to forcibly remove electrons from atoms (chiefly electrons and photons for this discussion).

Electron Volt (eV). A unit of kinetic energy, equivalent to that acquired by an electron when accelerated by a potential of 1 volt. A photon has kinetic energy which can be measured in eV; a photon of red light has an energy of about 1.8 eV; one of blue light, about 3 eV; and a photon emitted by a ^{99m}Tc nucleus can have an energy of 140,000 eV (140 *keV*).

Kiloelectron Volt (keV). 1000 electron volts (eV)

Megaelectron Volt (MeV). 1 million electron volts (eV)

Charge. Electrical charge, with the electron as a fundamental unit 1.6×10^{19} electrons = 1 coulomb (C). An average of 1.6×10^{19} electrons flowing past a point in 1 second is a current of 1 ampere (A).

Current.   Movement of charge (electrons) past a point. Electrons moving past a point at a rate of 6.25×10^{18} per second = 1 ampere, or at a rate of 6.25×10^{12} per second = 1 microampere (μA).

Counting.   A jargon word meaning the detection of ionizing radiation entities (particles or photons) as discrete events, and including the recording of the resulting *voltage pulses* by simple totalizing in a *scaler,* by a *count rate meter,* or by accumulating them in an image.

Voltage Pulse.   A sudden transient excursion of voltage, departing from some average or quiescent value to achieve a maximum departure and return; the use of "pulse" is not unlike that used to describe a transient excursion of arterial pressure felt in the human wrist. The voltage pulses we are concerned with last from a fraction of a microsecond to several hundred microseconds.

Scaler.   A totalizing device for accumulating voltage pulses resulting from detection of ionizing radiation entities or particles. The term is often used incorrectly to denote an entire counting system, including not only the totalizing register but also the high-voltage supply for a *Geiger tube* or *scintillation counter* and other auxiliary electronic circuits as well. The accumulated "count" is usually indicated by illuminated numerals.

Ratemeter (or "Count Rate Meter").   A device serving in lieu of, or in conjunction with, a scaler that indicates the average number of input *voltage pulses* (or "counts") over a prechosen time. The indication is continuous, may be observed by eye, or may be recorded on a strip-chart recorder to provide a record of counting rate versus time.

High-Voltage Supply.   The polarizing voltage applied to *gas-filled detectors* to facilitate the collection of electrons and form the output current or the output voltage pulse. Also the source of the successive accelerating voltages for the dynodes and anode of a *photomultiplier tube* resulting in the multiplication and collection of electrons from a radiation detection event in the *scintillation crystal.*

Gas-filled Detector.   A radiation detecting device, operating on the principle that ionizing radiation can be detected by collecting the electrons and positive ions liberated in a gaseous medium between two electrodes operated with an electric field between them. *Ionization chambers, proportional counters,* and *Geiger-Müller* counters are examples of gas-filled detectors.

Ionization Chamber.   A particular configuration of gas-filled detector, operated so that the charge gathered by the collecting electrodes (and, hence, the total output current) consists of the ions liberated by the advent of ionizing radiation. With no ionization, no current flows.

Proportional Counter.   An ionization chamber operated with a much higher electric field between the collecting electrodes. Electrons liberated by ionization are quickly accelerated and acquire enough energy to cause more ionization. The result is a multiplication of the original ionization, which is much easier to measure because it is larger and which provides a measure of particle or photon energy because it is proportional to the original ionization.

Geiger-Müller Counter.   Often called a "Geiger tube" or a Geiger counter; a gas-filled detector operated with an extremely high electric field between its electrodes.

Electrons liberated by ionization are violently accelerated toward the collecting electrodes causing a subsequent cascade of ionization so that essentially all of the gas in the device is ionized. This, in turn, results in a rapid collection of a large charge, which is converted into a large voltage pulse. This voltage pulse is formed for each detected particle and is independent of particle energy.

Valence Band.   The designation for the highest bands of energies normally occupied by electrons in atoms which are grouped together in large numbers. Electrons in the valence bands normally account for interactions between atoms.

Conduction Band.   The next allowed energy band above the valence band of atoms. Electrons in the conduction bands are shared between all atoms in a grouping and are free to wander from atom to atom. Coherent movement of electrons in the conduction bands constitutes electrical current through the matter.

Semiconductor.   A type of matter that is neither an electrical conductor (in which there is an overlap of the valence and conduction bands) nor an insulator (in which there is a large energy gap between the valence and conduction bands). The difference between an insulator and a semiconductor is that in the former the energy gap is so large that heat excitation of electrons from the valence band to the conduction band is unlikely, whereas in the latter considerable heat excitation of electrons into the conduction band occurs. The elements silicon and germanium are semiconductors.

"Hole."   A vacancy in the valence band of atoms. Holes are created when electrons are excited from the valence band to the conduction band. These vacancies, or holes, are able to move from atom to atom and their movement constitutes current.

Carrier.   A carrier of charge. Electrons are carriers of negative charge and holes effectively are carriers of positive charge.

n-Type Semiconductor.   A semiconductor material made with impurities that introduce electrons into the conduction bands independent of thermal excitation. Such material becomes electron conducting.

p-Type Semiconductor.   A semiconductor material made with impurities that introduces holes into the valence bands independent of thermal excitation. Such material becomes hole conducting.

Ohmic Contact.   An electrical contact to a semiconductor material which does not disturb the internal carrier concentration of the semiconductor. For example, if two such contacts are attached to a semiconductor material and if an electron is removed via one contact, the other contact injects an electron to replace the departed one.

p-n Junction.   A physical contact between a p-type semiconductor and n-type material. This is a "blocking" type contact that prevents the injection of an electron (or hole) from the opposite contact. Thus, by means of a p-n junction, both electrons and holes can be extracted from semiconductor materials, leaving them "depleted."

Intrinsic Semiconductor Material.   A semiconductor material that is ideally free of thermal excitation or impurities that cause excess carrier populations and thus exhibits low conductivity (high resistivity). As impurity-free material essentially does not exist, controlled introduction of carrier-donor materials have been used to compensate for excess carrier populations. "Lithium-compensated" low-resistivity p-type material exhibits a resistivity comparable with true intrinsic material.

Depletion Region. That portion of a piece of semiconductor material from which electrons have been removed from the conduction bands and from which holes have been removed from the valence bands. Such a region is formed by extraction of the carriers by use of blocking contacts and externally applied voltages. Intrinsic, or i-type, material can serve as a sort of permanent "depletion region," because of its lack of carrier population.

Semiconductor Detector. A type of radiation detector employing semiconductor materials. One type is the "surface barrier detector," which is a p-n junction made by the formation of a strongly p-type surface on a block of n-type silicon or germanium. Another is the "lithium-drifted detector," which consists of a block of lithium-compensated material between p-type and n-type electrodes.

Scintillation Counter. A radiation detection device consisting of a scintillation crystal coupled to a photomultiplier tube.

Scintillation Crystal. A monocrystal of some material that produces light scintillations when it absorbs ionizing radiation. The crystal used almost exclusively in nuclear medicine is sodium iodide (kin to sodium chloride, or rock salt) activated with a pinch of the element, thallium. It is abbreviated as NaI(Tl).

Photomultiplier Tube. A device that receives energy in the form of light photons, initially producing a number of electrons proportional to total light energy; it then accelerates these electrons so that they smash successively into a number of surfaces (called "dynodes") so as to dislodge more than their original number of electrons; these, too, enter the stream and all are collected at the "anode." For every original electron produced in the original light-to-electron conversion of energy, as many as 100,000 or even a million or more may be collected at the anode.

Scintillation Probe. An assembly, usually consisting of a scintillation crystal, a photomultiplier tube (which comprises a scintillation counter) in a suitable housing for mounting from a support, and fitted with some kind of collimator. Scintillation probes may be handheld or machine mounted, as in rectilinear scanners.

Energy-selective Counting System. A radiation detection system consisting of a radiation detector whose output is proportional to energy deposited in a detector by an ionizing radiation entity or particle, and which can be sorted out with a pulse height analyzer so that, in effect, detected radiation can be recorded or rejected depending on its energy. This system would embody either a scintillation counter or a semiconductor detector.

Preamplifier. The "front end," or input component of a linear amplifier, usually mounted physically close to a radiation detector. Its function is to provide power amplification to drive the detector signal through a cable to the principal part of the *linear amplifier.*

Linear Amplifier. A device to magnify the output of a scintillation counter so that its output voltage pulse has a maximum amplitude proportional to the total charge collected at the anode of the photomultiplier tube. The output of the linear amplifier is examined by the *pulse height analyzer* in an energy-selective counting system.

Threshold.   The name for the level to which a voltage pulse must rise to be detectable to a discriminator.

Discriminator.   An electrical circuit that functions as a "go-no-go" gauge for voltage pulses. Those pulses that exceed a certain threshold are announced by an output pulse (usually of constant size and shape) from the discriminator, which can drive scalers and ratemeters.

Pulse-Height Analyzer.   A device, usually consisting of two or more discriminators together with some auxiliary electronic circuits, designed to produce an output when the threshold of one discriminator but *not* the higher threshold of the other discriminator has been exceeded by a voltage pulse. This is the heart of any energy-selective counting system and is the means by which the voltage pulses from some detection events are recorded to the exclusion of others. Also drives scalers, ratemeters, and the like.

Rectilinear Scanner.   Consists of a machine-mounted scintillation counter, fitted with a *focused collimator* (making a directional scintillation probe) that is moved back and forth systematically over a subject, coupled to a *photorecorder* that makes, by means of a light source flashing at a photographic film, a radioactivity map of the subject. Usually the subject is emitting gamma rays, which are detected by the scintillation probe.

Scintillation Camera.   A device for imaging a gamma-ray emitting subject that uses a large, disc-shaped scintillation crystal. By electronic means, a flash of light is made to appear on the face of a *cathode ray tube* at a position corresponding to the position on the scintillation crystal that a gamma ray was absorbed.

Collimator.   A device, usually thick and sievelike, used to restrict the direction by which a gamma ray may enter a scintillation crystal. Scintillation cameras often use collimators of parallel, constant-diameter, straight holes in a block of lead. Rectilinear scanners, on the other hand, usually make use of a *focused collimator*. Scintillation cameras also may use a *pinhole collimator*.

Focused Collimator.   A collimator made of tapering round or hexagonal holes in a block of lead, constructed such that the holes are (usually) aimed at a common point. These holes are usually grouped in a circularly symmetric pattern around a common central axis.

Photorecorder.   A plotting device, moving in synchronism, with the scintillation probe of a rectilinear scanner that exposes a photographic film to a light source that flashes with each gamma-ray detection event accepted by the pulse-height analyzer (or at a rate proportional to the counting, or detection, rate).

Cathode Ray Tube (CRT).   A display device, not unlike a television picture tube, in which an electron stream is directed from an "electron gun" to smash into a phosphor (a substance that glows when impacted by energetic electrons). The electron stream can be deflected up and down and left and right and can be turned on and off (like the stream from a garden hose). By this means, flashes of light can be made to appear on the face (phosphor) of the CRT each time an acceptable gamma-ray detection event occurs in the scintillation crystal of a scintillation camera. A time photographic exposure of the face of the CRT builds up the scintillation camera image.

Pinhole Collimator.   A single-aperture collimator, usually mounted several inches in front of the scintillation crystal of a scintillation camera so that, in the manner of Leonardo da Vinci's "camera obscura," an image of the object space on the opposite side of the aperture appears on the crystal. This system operates exactly like a pinhole camera for light, except that its "light" consists of gamma rays emitted by objects in the object space.

BASIC RADIATION DETECTION DEVICES AND SYSTEMS

Gas-filled Detectors

Almost any apparatus can be a "radiation detector" if it provides a means of measuring the electrical result of the encounter of ionizing radiation with the apparatus. One of the simplest is the "ionization chamber,"[1]* a gas-filled device (Fig. 1) that measures the amount of current that flows in an external circuit when ionization (i.e., electron liberation) takes place in the gas with which it is filled within its volume. The filling gas may be any of several, even air. The device is operated with an externally applied voltage such that the liberated electrons are completely collected without loss due to recombination (to form neutral atoms) or without multiplication (secondary ionization due to the collection process). Thus the current circulating through the chamber and voltage supply is quantitatively indicative of the radiation flux through the chamber.

The ionization chamber is limited to measurements of radiation flux, requiring a steady exposure to a radiation source to establish a measurable output current. These currents are quite small, making the ionization chamber a relatively "insensitive" device that is most useful for measuring radiation from intense sources. Other detectors to be described are poorly suited for measurements of intense sources because they detect and report individual particles or photons and thus are of relatively high sensitivity.

Gas-filled detectors can be operated with a much higher electric field between electrodes than is used in the ionization chamber with the result that electrons are accelerated in the collection process to the extent that they have sufficient energy to ionize other atoms with which they collide. The secondary ionization produces electrons that produce tertiary ionization and so on. Thus the original ionization current is multiplied to a much larger value which is easier to form into a small voltage pulse that serves as an announcement that an individual radiation entity has been detected. Moreover, the height of the voltage pulse is proportional to the amount of original ionization produced in the chamber, which in turn is proportional to the energy lost by the radiation entity in the detector. Thus, this device is called a proportional counter.

Proportional counters are useful for energy-selective counting of x-rays and gamma rays in the low-energy (5–100 keV) region; prior to the advent of scintillation counters, they were the only means of such detection. Gas-filled proportional counters are not used to any substantial extent in nuclear medicine today.

A Geiger-Müller (G-M) counter[2] is a gas-filled detector operated with very high electric fields caused by high ($\sim$900 V) accelerating voltages and a very thin wire as a collecting electrode. Current in the absence of ionization in the device is very low because of a very low ($\sim\frac{1}{75}$ atm) gas pressure. When an entering particle or photon initiates ionization, an action similar to that in a proportional counter takes place, ex-

---

* Reference 1 is recommended to the reader for a readable, yet competent treatment of ionization chambers and semiconductor detectors. The simple language and analogies make its reading rewarding to those with a minimum of background knowledge.

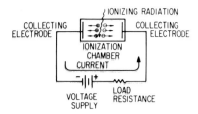

Fig. 1. A simple ionization chamber. Incoming radiation ionizes the gas atoms or molecules within the chamber. The liberated electrons are collected by the positive electrode, thus constituting a current in the circuit. The output indication usually is measured by means of the voltage produced across the load resistance by the passage of the current.

cept that the multiplication is so large that virtually all of the gas in the chamber becomes ionized. This results in a very large output voltage pulse which is of the same height for each initiating event (at a given applied voltage). This constant-size pulse, independent of the energy of the particle or photon that caused it, makes subsequent electronic handling and recording of the event relatively simple. Figure 2 illustrates the simple nature of a Geiger-Müller counter system.

The height of the voltage pulse from a G-M counter is a strong function of the applied voltage. Because all the pulses are about the same size, however, a "plateau" of counting rate *versus* applied voltage exists above the value of applied high voltage that causes the output pulses to exceed the input threshold of the recording device (the scaler in Fig. 2). This is illustrated in Fig. 3. Where the plateau is as flat as it is in Fig. 3, the counting rate is quite independent of applied voltage which reduces the performance requirements of the voltage supply and reduces criticality of adjustment. Actual plateaus are seldom as flat as that in Fig. 3, however, as the output pulses are not really of exactly the same size. There are always some undersize pulses produced, particularly in oddly shaped chambers, and increases of applied voltage boosts these substandard pulses over the scaler input threshold.

Special, small-size versions of the G-M counter are used for beta particle detection in body cavities[2] and at surgery. One such use is for detection of beta particles from ^{32}P in the identification of intraocular melanomas.[3, 4] This use will be discussed in a subsequent chapter, along with the competitive semiconductor ocular detector.

Semiconductor Detectors[1, 5]

At first glance, using a solid instead of a gas in an ionization chamber would appear to have at least two desirable attributes. First, the solid is far more likely to stop, and absorb the energy of, particles and photons. Second, the average energy required to produce one unit of ionization (electron-positive ion pair) in a gas is around 30 eV; in a solid, the energy required to liberate an electron and produce an electron vacancy (electron-hole pair) is around 3 eV. Therefore, ionizing radiation produces about 10 times as many charge carriers in a solid as in a gas. This simplifies amplification problems and improves the statistical variation in the charge produced from identical events.

A semiconductor counter similar to the ionization chamber in Fig. 1 could be constructed with a bar of semiconductor material between two ohmic contacts serving as collecting electrodes. Such a counter is illustrated in Fig. 4.[1] Incoming radiation would create electron-hole pairs; the electrons would migrate (with energies in the conduction band) to the positive (ohmic) collecting electrode. The vacancies in the valence band (holes) would migrate to the negative electrode. This device, therefore, would more properly be called a "conductivity" counter rather than a "solid ionization chamber."

Such a device would be useless, however, because a large number of electron-hole

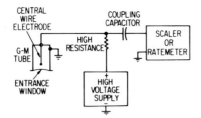

Fig. 2. A simple Geiger-Müller (G-M) counting system. Each particle of incoming radiation causes essentially all of the gas in the tube to become quickly ionized. The rapid collection of the charge on the central wire electrode causes a high current to flow for a brief time in the high resistance connected to the high voltage supply. This develops a pulse that is used to actuate the scaler or ratemeter. The simplicity of this system is one of its advantages.

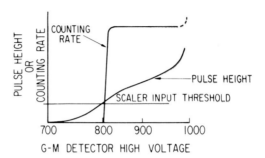

Fig. 3. Curves of pulse height and associated counting rate *versus* G-M detector high voltage, with a radiation source of constant intensity. Virtually all output pulses from a G-M tube have the same height, and their height increases rapidly with applied high voltage. When these pulses are below the scaler input threshold, there is no counting rate; after the pulses have achieved a height equal to the threshold, raising the applied voltage increases only their size and not their number, hence counting rates are constant with applied voltage. This flat response of counting rate with high voltage is called a "plateau."

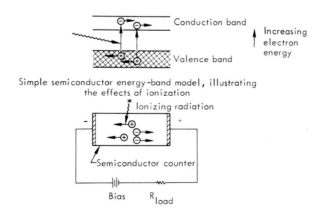

Fig. 4. A simple semiconductor conductivity counter. This is analogous to the ionization chamber of Fig. 1, with the semiconductor material taking the place of the filling gas. Incoming radiation creates electron-hole pairs, with the electrons being lifted to energies in the conduction band and leaving holes in the valence band. This is shown for illustrative purposes only, as thermally generated currents would completely swamp any ionization currents in an actual device. Reprinted by permission from reference 1.

pairs would be thermally generated (largely from impurities in the material), causing a background current that would be orders of magnitude greater than any additional current produced by ionizing radiation. In effect, the thermal background current ruins the counter. An extremely pure semiconductor material would be sufficiently free of thermally excited electron-hole pairs, but such material, for practical purposes, is unavailable.

Fortunately, there is a better way to realize the advantages postulated for the solid counter over the gas ionization chamber. The detector may be constructed using a p-n junction, to take advantage of the properties of physical contact between p-type (hole-conducting) and n-type (electron-conducting) semiconductor materials. A p-n junction may be formed by a variety of processes. One such is illustrated in Fig. 5,[5] where a strongly p-type surface is formed on n-type silicon. When a voltage is applied as shown, electrons will be extracted from the n-type region nearest the p-type layer, without electrons being injected from the p-type material. Thus, there is formed a "depletion region," and because of the removal of carriers, background currents are acceptably small.

When radiation enters (through the p-type surface barrier) electron-hole pairs are formed in the depletion region. The collection of this charge forms a voltage pulse that may be amplified for analysis and recording, and which is directly proportional to the energy absorbed in the depletion region.

Silicon surface barrier detectors (Fig. 5) may be operated at room temperature, whereas germanium surface barrier detectors must be operated at greatly reduced temperature, usually 77°K (liquid nitrogen). Silicon, because of its low atomic number and modest density, absorbs gamma and x-ray photons poorly. As a result, it is more useful for detecting charged particles (beta particles, specifically for medical applications).

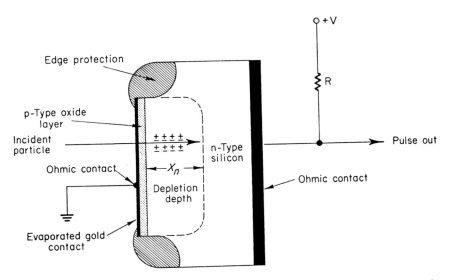

Fig. 5. A surface-barrier semiconductor detector, utilizing a p-n junction. When the detector has voltage applied (biased) as shown, electrons (majority carrier in n-type silicon) are removed from the region immediately adjacent to the p-type material. This depleted region becomes the active volume of the detector. Reprinted by permission from reference 5.

Another approach that effectively creates larger depletion regions (and, hence, larger response to ionizing radiation) is illustrated in Fig. 6.[5] By drifting lithium into p-type material while applying a voltage and high ambient temperatures, a region is created wherein the excess carriers (holes) are compensated by electrons donated by the lithium atoms. The result is an ersatz semiconductor that behaves as if it were quite pure, with greatly reduced thermally generated carriers. This technique of fabrication of essentially intrinsic semiconductor material is called "lithium compensation."

Lithium-drifted detectors achieve large depletion regions more easily than p-n junction detectors and, as a result, are in more widespread use, especially in larger sizes. Lithium-drifted silicon is abbreviated SiLi, which colloquially is pronounced "silly." Lithium-compensated germanium detectors are denoted GeLi, pronounced "jelly."

The former have poor efficiency for detection of photons, good efficiency for detecting charged particles (electrons or beta particles), and are stable at room temperature. These detectors are in prevalent use for detection of beta particles in identification of intraocular melanomas (to be described in a subsequent chapter). The GeLi detectors, on the other hand, detect gamma and x-ray photons with better efficiency and very good energy resolution, but must be operated at very low (liquid nitrogen) temperatures. It is chiefly for this reason (and that of cost) that the GeLi detector has not yet come into widespread nuclear medical use.

Scintillation Detectors

Gas-filled detectors have poor efficiencies for detection of gamma and x-ray photons. At present, semiconductor detectors are limited to relatively small sizes and used mostly for particle detection. Though their use is required in specialized applications,[6] effective and practical nuclear medicine procedures require the maximum efficiency for external de-

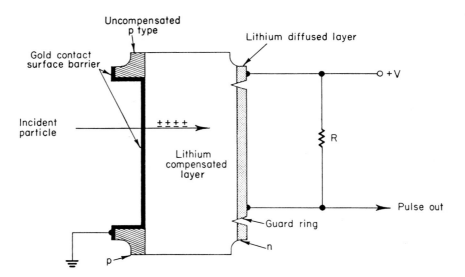

Fig. 6. A lithium-drifted detector. The lithium-compensated layer has its excess carriers neutralized and thus serves as a large "depletion region" for the detector. Reprinted by permission from reference 5.

tection of gamma rays in vivo. Additionally, imaging procedures require energy discrimination as well.

The requirements of efficiency and of energy discrimination have led to the widespread use of a solid proportional counter that scintillates with an energy proportional to the gamma or x-ray energy absorbed. This device is called a "scintillation counter."[7] Where the material is sodium iodide activated with a trace of thallium—NaI(Tl)—the scintillation counter has an almost linearly proportional energy response, has high detection efficiency and can be made in very large sizes. The energy-selective capability of a NaI(Tl) scintillation counter is not nearly as good as that of the GeLi detector, in that it produces very broad spectral distributions from monoenergetic gamma rays (Fig. 7). Despite this disadvantage, it is the most practical gamma ray detector and is in overwhelmingly prevalent use in nuclear medicine for external detection of in vivo radioactivity.

In scintillation detectors (and in semiconductor detectors, too), the energy of a "detected" particle or gamma ray is converted into a charge (number of electrons) proportional to that energy. The charge is, in turn, converted to a voltage pulse whose height is proportional to the gamma energy absorbed in the NaI(Tl) scintillation crystal. This process is illustrated in Fig. 8. The purpose of the photomultiplier tube is to convert the feeble scintillations emanating from the crystal (in response to "detection" of a gamma ray) into an electrically significant and usable bundle of charge. The charge-to-voltage (pulse height) is accomplished in the electronic circuits associated with the scintillation detector (and semiconductor detector).

ENERGY-SELECTIVE COUNTING SYSTEMS

Simple Systems

The simplicity of a system using a G-M detector was shown in Fig. 3 and derives from the energy-independent output from the G-M tube itself.

Energy-selective counting systems are necessarily more complicated. A complete system for a scintillation detector is shown in Fig. 9a, and for a semiconductor detector in Fig. 9b, which is offered chiefly to indicate a basic similarity. This structure is generally common to all applications of gamma ray counting with NaI(Tl). The widest variations take place in the "recording or indicating means," which for thyroid uptake studies and test-tube-sample counting may be a scaler. For a similarly simple system for measuring renal radioactivity as a function of time, the recording means might be a ratemeter coupled to a strip-chart recorder. For imaging applications, the recording means may be a device for making on photographic film an "activity map" of the subject.

The function of the linear amplifier is to generate a voltage pulse proportional to the charge arriving from the detector by way of the preamplifier. The heights of the pulses from the linear amplifier are examined by a pulse-height analyzer (or threshold discriminator) which provides an output pulse for each input pulse in a prescribed pulse height interval (or above a given threshold).

As the pulse heights are proportional to gamma ray energy, this has the effect of "tuning" the system to accept only gamma rays of certain energies. This is helpful in eliminating from the measurement (or image) those gamma rays that are scattered

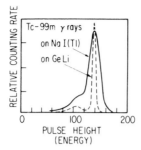

Fig. 7. Comparative pulse heights spectra from a sodium iodide scintillation detector and a lithium-drifted germanium semiconductor detector. The "line-width" of the semiconductor detector is much narrower making it a better energy-selective detector. There are, however, reasons why it is not in common use in nuclear medicine. Semiconductor detectors also show excellent energy resolution with charged particles, such as electrons.

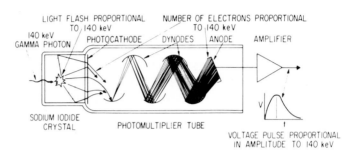

Fig. 8. A schematic representation of a scintillation detector. Light is emitted by the scintillation crystal proportional to the amount of gamma ray energy absorbed by the crystal. The light in turn excites electrons from the photocathode of the photomultiplier tube. These original electrons are multiplied from 100,000 to 1 million times in the photomultiplier. The output current is converted to a voltage pulse which will be proportional in its amplitude to the energy deposited in the crystal.

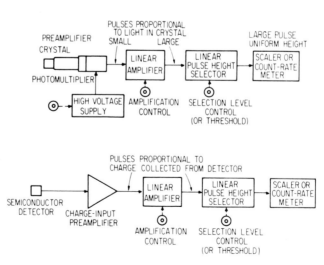

Fig. 9. Energy-selective counting systems using a scintillation detector (a) and a semiconductor detector (b). The two systems are essentially the same with the exception that the photomultiplier tube operates with a high voltage of from 750–1500 V, whereas the semiconductor detector operates with very low voltages supplied by the preamplifier.

before they leave the subject (or patient). Scattered gamma rays seem to originate at the scattering site—not their true origin—but lose some energy in the process. Thus "tuning in" on unscattered (or full-energy) gamma photons makes a cleaner measurement.[8] The output of the pulse-height analyzer (or discriminator) drives the "recording or indicating means."

More Complex Systems—Imaging

A radioactivity map of a subject may be made by use of a scintillation probe moved about by a rectilinear scanner or by a large-diameter scintillation crystal in a scintillation camera.

The rectilinear scanner (Fig. 10) moves a scintillation detector equipped with a directionalizing focused collimator in a systematic to-and-fro manner over the subject. Moving in synchronism with the detector is an impulse-type indicator, usually a pulsed light source moving over a piece of x-ray film, that flashes each time a count is accepted and passed by the pulse-height analyzer. This pulsed plotting device is called a photorecorder.

Rectilinear scanners are in common use for many body organ systems. Hence, they are capable of scanning large areas (14 in. × 17 in.) up to total-body areas (24 in. × 72 in.). Where the area of the scan exceeds the area of the usual 14 in. × 17 in. film reduced recording formats (minification) are provided. Dual detecting probes (usually

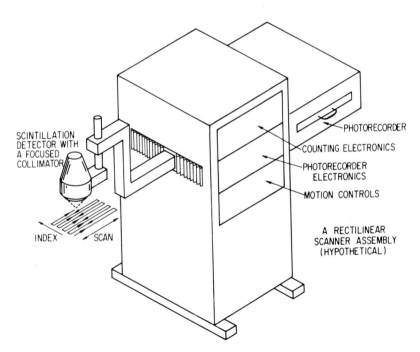

Fig. 10. A representation of the structure of a rectilinear scanner. As the scintillation detector with its focused collimator is moved back and forth in a rectilinear raster, a light source is moving over a film in the photorecorder with a motion corresponding to that of the detector. As activity is detected, a pulsed light source exposes the film at a location corresponding to that of the activity.

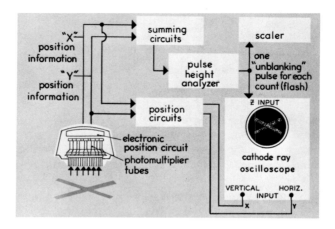

Fig. 11. A schematic representation of an Anger scintillation camera. For each scintillation event, a pair of pulses each representing the *x* and *y* coordinates of the event are sent to the display device, a cathode ray oscilloscope. The position pulses also are summed into a common pulse, representative of the total amount of light produced by the scintillator. This pulse is subjected to pulse height analysis and if accepted causes a flash of light to appear on the face of the cathode ray oscilloscope at a position determined by the position pulses. A photographic camera with its shutter open integrates these events into a meaningful image.

synchronized, opposed over-and-under arrangements) provide two images with one positioning of the subject and materially reduce examination time.

Of possible interest in nuclear ophthalmic applications is the fact that where gamma ray energies are low (28 keV from iodine-125 up to 140 keV from technetium-99m) and where the subject is small (e.g., a thyroid gland or an eyeball), specialized rectilinear scanners for these conditions are quite feasible. Such are not commercially available at this time, however. Detailed imaging of the orbit with iodine-125 labeled compounds would require such a device, as conventional rectilinear scanners may be awkward to use and generally do not provide adequate spatial resolution. In addition, the scintillation camera is unsuitable for use with very low (28 keV) gamma ray energies.

Scintillation cameras are useful for making static images somewhat more rapidly than with single-probe rectilinear scanners because of the larger detector area. (Figs. 11 and 12). Because only the scintillation camera is able to view an entire organ at once, it is required when dynamic, or time-sequence, studies are to be made. The arrangement by which an image, formed by gamma photons arriving at specific locations on the scintillation crystal, is presented on a display cathode ray tube is shown in Fig. 11.[9]

Because of statistical limitations in the detection process, there is uncertainty (from event to event) in the X and Y positional signal pulses. As a result, a scintillation

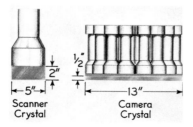

Scanner
Crystal

Camera
Crystal

Fig. 12. Typical detector sizes for rectilinear scanners and for scintillation cameras. The areas of the fields of visions of scintillation cameras typically are four to five times that for rectilinear scanners. Rectilinear scanners, however, may have two detectors operating simultaneously. In typical studies, total procedure times tend to be about the same. Reprinted by permission from reference 8.

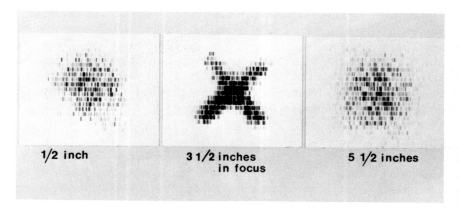

1/2 inch   3 1/2 inches   5 1/2 inches
                   in focus

Fig. 13. Images of blotting paper crosses soaked with cobalt-57 and mounted at varying distances from the face of a focused collimator. Only the image that was in the focal plane of the collimator was imaged recognizably. All images, however, contain about the same number of counts. Thus, it is seen that a focused collimator is crudely tomographic in its operation. Reprinted by permission from reference 8.

camera image of a point source is not a point but rather a blur that might be as large as a centimeter across. Thus the camera has an inherent resolution loss that has no exact counterpart in the rectilinear scanner. With this exception, however, image detail with both cameras and scanners is limited by the geometric properties of the collimators used.

Rectilinear scanners use focused collimators chiefly to achieve high geometric detection efficiency through the use of large-diameter scintillation crystals. A sort of tomographic effect is (not deliberately) achieved by the common aiming of the collimating channels. The result is that the only detailed structures appearing in the image are in the focal plane (usually about 6–10 cm from the collimator) when the object was scanned. (Fig. 13).[8]

Scintillation cameras, on the other hand, usually employ collimators made of straight, parallel channels in lead. With these collimators, image detail is best when the collimator is in contact with the subject. Subjects greater than 15 cm from the collimator will show extremely poor image detail.

Another collimator in use with the scintillation camera consists of a single aperture in a tungsten block, mounted in a shielding cone 15–20 cm from the crystal (Fig. 14).[10] This "pinhole" collimator derives from the pinhole camera and is of interest in nuclear ophthalmology because it can provide an enlarged image of small subjects. The basic spatial resolving property of a pinhole collimator is, of course, determined by the size of the aperture, usually 4.5–7 mm; counting rates usually vary with the *area* of the aperture. This collimator has a useful characteristic in that as the subject is brought closer to

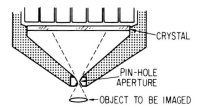

CRYSTAL

PIN-HOLE
APERTURE

OBJECT TO BE IMAGED

Fig. 14. A longitudinal section of a scintillation camera with a pinhole collimator attached. When the object to be imaged is placed closer to the pinhole than the aperture-to-crystal distance, the image is magnified. A magnified image helps to diminish the effect of the camera's intrinsic blurring of the image.

the aperture, counting rates rise and the image is magnified. The magnified image tends to diminish the effect of the inherent resolution problem of the camera mentioned earlier.

A special "micropinhole" collimator provides the necessary spatial resolution to perform lacrimal duct patency studies with ^{99m}Tc pertechnetate.[11] The loss of sensitivity with the small (1.1 mm) aperture is not significant because even small (100 μCi) drops of ^{99m}Tc pertechnetate provide satisfactory counting rates.

SUMMARY

The application of nuclear medical techniques to ophthalmologic problems heretofore has been limited. There is, therefore, the likelihood that the ophthalmologist has had limited opportunity to become familiar with the hardware used in nuclear medicine methodology. This presentation has been directed toward the beginning of the removal of that impediment. Accordingly, it is not a complete, all-encompassing treatment; rather, it has been designed to provide the ophthalmologist with a grasp of operating schema and a lexicon of terms to use wherever the application of nuclear medical instruments to his specialty is discussed.

REFERENCES

1. Armantrout, G. A.: Principles of Semiconductor Detector Operation. In Hoffer, P. B., Beck, R. N., and Gottschalk, A., Eds., *Semiconductor Detectors in the Future of Nuclear Medicine,* The Society of Nuclear Medicine, New York, 1971.

2. Robinson, C. V.: Geiger-Muller and Proportional Counters. In Hine, G. J., Ed., *Instrumentation in Nuclear Medicine,* Academic Press, New York, 1967.

3. Thomas, C. I., Krohmer, J. S., and Storaasli, J. P.: Detection of Intraocular Tumors with Radioactive Phosphorus. A Preliminary Report with Special Reference to Differentiation of Cause of Retinal Separation, *Arch. Ophthalmol.* **47**:276 (1952).

4. Carmichael, P. L., Holst, G. C., Federman, J. L., and Shields, J. A.: The Present Status of the ^{32}P Test in Ophthalmology. In Croll, M. N., Brady, L. W., Honda, T., and Wallner, R. J., Eds., *New Techniques in Tumor Localization and Radioimmunoassay.* John Wiley, New York, 1974.

5. Friedland, S. S., and Zatzick, M. R.: Semiconductor Detectors. In Hine, G. J., Ed., *Instrumentation in Nuclear Medicine,* Academic Press, New York, 1967.

6. Hoffer, P. B., Bernstein, J., and Gottschalk, A.: Clinical Results in Fluorescent Scanning. In Hoffer, P. B., Beck, R. N., and Gottschalk, A., Eds., *Semiconductor Detectors in the Future of Nuclear Medicine,* The Society of Nuclear Medicine, New York, 1971.

7. Ross, D. A., and Harris, C. C.: Measurement of Radioactivity. In Wagner, H. N., Jr., Ed., *Principles of Nuclear Medicine,* W. B. Saunders, Philadelphia, 1968.

8. Harris, C. C.: Instrumentation Factors in Visualization of Tumors. In Croll, M. N., Brady, L. W., Honda, T., and Wallner, R. J., Eds., *New Techniques in Tumor Localization and Radioimmunoassay,* John Wiley, New York, 1974.

9. Harris, C. C. Instrumentation: Imaging Devices. An Audio/Visual Program in Nuclear Medicine, Blaufox, M.D., and Freeman, L. M., Eds., Nuclear Associates, Inc., Westbury, N.Y., 1974.

10. Anger, H. O.: Sensitivity and Resolution of the Scintillation Camera. In Gottschalk, A., and Beck, R. N., Eds., *Fundamental Problems in Scanning,* Charles C. Thomas, Springfield, Ill., 1968.

11. Rossomundo, R. M., Carlton, W. H., Trueblood, J. H., and Thomas, R. P.: A New Method of Evaluating Lacrimal Drainage. *Arch. Ophthalmol.* **88**:523 (1972).

Radiopharmaceuticals in Nuclear Ophthalmology

Gerald A. Bruno, Ph.D.
Director,
Diagnostic Research and
Development Department,
The Squibb Institute for
Medical Research,
New Brunswick, New Jersey

Along with nuclear instrumentation, radiopharmaceuticals play a key role in the application of nuclear diagnostic procedures to ophthalmology. Basic to an understanding of these techniques is a knowledge of the physical and chemical properties of the commonly used radionuclides and the biological behavior of the compounds to which these radionuclides are attached.

The following information is intended as a basic review of the physics, chemistry, and biology of radionuclides of importance in nuclear ophthalmology. Hopefully, it will provide the nonnuclear scientist with an adequate foundation to appreciate the role of radionuclides in diagnostic ophthalmology.

PHOSPHORUS-32

Physical Properties

Phosphorus-32 (^{32}P) is one of the oldest radionuclides used in medicine today. It is produced in a nuclear reactor via the nuclear transmutation reaction

$$^{32}S(n,p)^{32}P$$

In actual practice, a stable or nonradioactive source of sulfur is placed in the high neutron flux of a nuclear reactor, where the nucleus of the sulfur atom captures a neutron and expels a proton. Because the resulting nuclear configuration is unnatural, the nucleus is unstable, and the element formed (^{32}P) is said to be radioactive. The emission of atomic particles or energy, in the quest to achieve stability, is the radioactivity that is utilized in the medical applications of ^{32}P.

Before discussing the types of radiation emitted by radioactive elements, it is important to understand the relatively simple concept of radioactive half-life (T½) that defines the rate at which a radionuclide decays, or returns to stability. A radionuclide with a highly unstable nuclear configuration will decay very rapidly, in a matter of seconds, minutes, or days, while the more stable configurations will decay over a period of years or even millions of years. The radioactive T½ of ^{32}P is 14.3 days, which means that one-half of the unstable nuclei will revert to a stable form in a period of 14.3 days. For example, if we have 1000 radioactive atoms of ^{32}P, at the end of 14.3 days, only 500 atoms of ^{32}P will remain. In the next 14.3 day period, 50% of the remaining radioactive atoms will decay, and 250 ^{32}P atoms will remain at 28.6 days. At 42.9 days, only 125 atoms of ^{32}P will remain. While it is obvious that radioactive decay is exponential, for practical purposes it is generally assumed that a radioactive element will undergo complete decay in a period of 10 half-lives.

The three types of radiation emitted in the decay of radionuclides are alpha (α), beta (β), and gamma (γ). Only the β and γ decay are important in nuclear ophthalmology and will be discussed further. Phosphorus-32 decays by beta or negatron emission, through a process that involves conversion of a neutron to a proton. The conversion is accomplished by the expulsion of a beta particle (β^- or negatron) from the nucleus, accompanied by a tiny atomic particle called a neutrino. The net effect of the decay is a drop in the energy level of the nucleus of 1.71 million electron volts (MeV). The nuclear changes associated with negatron emission from ^{32}P are depicted below.

$$\left(\begin{array}{c}15P\\17n\end{array}\right) \longrightarrow \left(\begin{array}{c}16P\\16N\end{array}\right) + \beta^- + \nu + 1.71 \text{ MeV}$$

$$^{32}_{15}P \qquad ^{32}_{16}S$$

Nucleus   Nucleus

The decay of ^{32}P can be summarized using a simplified version of the commonly employed nuclear decay scheme.

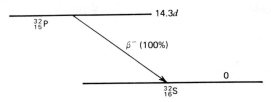

The β^- particles expelled from the ^{32}P nucleus are emitted with a continuous range of energies up to a maximum of 1.71 MeV. In accordance with the law of conservation of energy, the β^- particles that are emitted with less than the maximum 1.71 MeV energy, are accompanied by a neutrino. The neutrino has a mass of essentially zero and carries no electrical charge, but possesses momentum and energy. The energy of the neutrino that accompanies a β^- particle will be equal to the difference between the maximum 1.71 MeV energy and the energy of the β^- particle. This concept is graphically illustrated in Fig. 1.

The physical property that is of greatest importance in the medical application of radionuclides is the interaction of the emitted radiation with matter. The distance traveled by the emitted radiation in tissue will determine its utility in a variety of nuclear imaging procedures. The transmission of radiation through water provides a good approximation of tissue transmission and is depicted in Fig. 2. A 1 MeV α particle will travel only about 5 μ in water and thus cannot be used in nuclear imaging procedures. A 1 MeV β^- particle will travel up to 4 mm in water but is still not strong enough to be detected external to the body for most nuclear imaging procedures. Phosphorus-32 with a maximum energy of 1.71 MeV will travel up to 8.5 mm in water and thus can be detected when emanating from a body structure close to the surface, such as the eye. Because of reduced interaction with matter, the electromagnetic γ ray will travel long

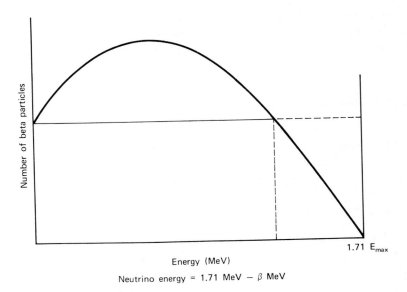

Neutrino energy = 1.71 MeV − β MeV

Fig. 1. ^{32}P beta particle spectrum.

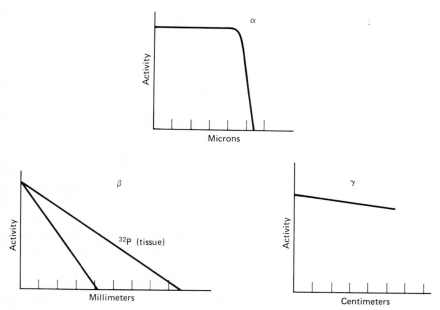

Fig. 2. Radiation transmission curves (1 MeV in water).

distances in water, and provide an effective means of imaging internal organs of the body. A 1 MeV γ ray is exponentially attenuated in water, falling to one-half of its original intensity at 20 cm.

Chemical Properties

Phosphorus-32 is generally made available in the simple chemical form of disodium phosphate (Na_2HPO_4). Pharmaceutical formulations are prepared by dissolving the radioactive material in water for injection, with a suitable preservative. Stable phosphate is usually added to the formulation in carrier amounts, and methyl and propyl parabens are commonly used as preservatives. Parenteral preparations can be sterilized by autoclaving or membrane filtration and are stable at room temperature.

Biological Properties

Phosphorus-32, as disodium phosphate, is handled by the body in the same manner as naturally occurring phosphorus (^{31}P) and participates in the general biochemical reactions of the body. Since all tissues of the body contain phosphorus, administration of radiophosphorus in readily ionizable form results in rapid distribution to all tissues. Tissues that utilize phosphorus in their metabolic processes take up the element more rapidly than others. Increased amounts of ^{32}P are incorporated in cells in which proliferation is most active, for example, the bone marrow. When mitosis is accelerated, the requirement for phosphorus is increased. Consequently, radioactive phosphorus will concentrate to a greater degree in cancerous cells than in noncancerous cells. This property provides the basis for application of ^{32}P to detection of ocular tumors.[1]

About 5 to 10% of the ^{32}P that is administered intravenously is excreted in the urine in the first 24 hours, and about 20% of the administered dose is excreted by the end of the first week. A very small percentage of the intravenously administered dose is found in the feces. Following oral administration, approximately 15 to 50% of the ^{32}P is excreted in the urine and feces during the first 4 to 6 days.[2]

TECHNETIUM-99m

Physical Properties

Technetium-99m (^{99m}Tc) is a relatively new radionuclide but has already become perhaps the most important radionuclide used in medicine today. The widespread acceptance of ^{99m}Tc for nuclear imaging procedures is based on its essentially ideal physical properties. These properties include a primary γ ray energy of 0.14 MeV, no β radiation, and a physical T½ of 6.1 hours. The 0.14 MeV γ energy is ideally suited to the gamma camera instrument systems and provides good penetration from deep-seated body organs, without significant penetration of the septa of the focusing collimators. The absence of β^- decay avoids unnecessary radiation dose to the patient from a source that adds nothing to the diagnostic information obtained. The 6.1 hour T½ also reduces the radiation dose to the patient by minimizing prolonged exposure to radiation after the diagnostic procedure has been completed. The reduced radiation dose associated with the use of ^{99m}Tc allows larger amounts of radioactivity to be safely administered to the patient, yielding images of greater resolution, more efficient utilization of expensive imaging equipment, and, when required, more frequent repetition of imaging procedures.

The 6.1 hour T½ of ^{99m}Tc, however, does create problems in the area of production and distribution of the radionuclide. Because distribution of 6.1 hour T½ ^{99m}Tc to all users is not practical, a device that has come to be known as the "radionuclide generator" has been developed to produce this invaluable nuclide.

In general, the radionuclide generator is composed of a longer lived "parent" nuclide, that decays to the shorter lived, medically useful "daughter" nuclide. The generator is constructed in such a way that the daughter nuclide can be easily separated or "milked" from the parent nuclide, leaving the parent behind to generate fresh daughter nuclide. The parent radionuclide used for ^{99m}Tc production is molybdenum-99 (^{99}Mo; T½ = 2.7 days). In the ^{99}Mo/^{99m}Tc generator, the ^{99}Mo is adsorbed on a bed of alumina, and after an appropriate decay interval, the ^{99m}Tc, as the pertechnetate (TcO$^-_4$), is separated from the ^{99}Mo by washing the alumina bed with physiological saline. Maximum amounts of ^{99m}Tc can be obtained from the generator by washing the alumina bed at 24-hour intervals. A diagram of the ^{99}Mo/^{99m}Tc generator is depicted in Fig. 3.

Technetium-99m is produced as a result of β^- decay of ^{99}Mo. The nucleus of the ^{99m}Tc is in a highly excited (metastable) state and rapidly decays to ^{99}Tc via a process referred to as isomeric transition. The simplified decay scheme is depicted below.

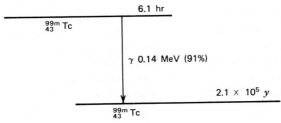

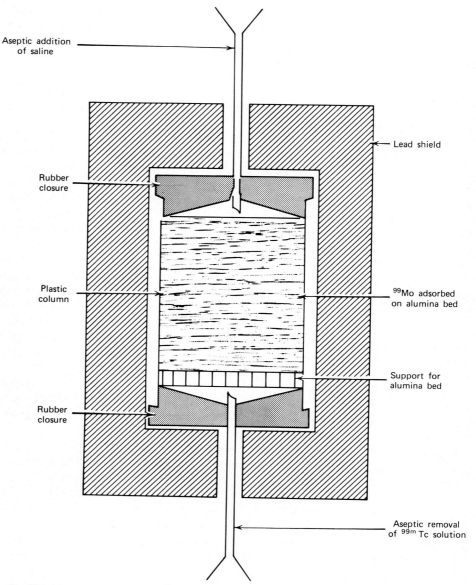

Fig. 3. ^{99}Mo/^{99m}Tc generator.

Chemical Properties

Technetium-99m is obtained from the ^{99}Mo/^{99m}Tc generator as the pertechnetate ion (TcO$_4^-$) in the +7 valence state. Sterile, nonpyrogenic solutions of ^{99m}Tc can be obtained from these generators, using aseptic techniques to introduce sterile, nonpyrogenic saline solution into the generator and to remove the ^{99m}Tc eluate. The pertechnetate solution can be used in a number of imaging procedures without chemical modification or can be used for tagging a variety of compounds for other imaging applications. To achieve binding of the ^{99m}Tc to other compounds, it is necessary to first reduce the ^{99m}Tc from the +7 to the +4 valence state, using reducing agents such as stannous (Sn^{++}) ion. Technetium-99m in the +4 valence state is highly reactive and has been successfully attached to a wide range of compounds of medical interest.

Because of the relatively short T½ of ^{99m}Tc, it is generally not necessary to include a preservative in its formulation.

Biological Properties

After intravenous administration, the blood disappearance curve of pertechnetate is biphasic, with an initial rapid phase and a subsequent slow phase. It has been suggested[3] that the rapid phase of pertechnetate disappearance from the blood represents equilibration with the interstitial fluid and localization in the stomach, thyroid, salivary glands, and extracellular space, and the slow phase represents urinary excretion and intracellular penetration. Estimates of the initial blood clearance half-time have ranged from 8 minutes to 1.5 hours, while estimates for the slower phase have ranged from 3 to 9 hours.[4]

Because of the rapid decay of ^{99m}Tc, excretion of pertechnetate has been measured in humans for only 72 hours. During the first 24 hours, excretion is rapid and almost entirely urinary. Subsequently, urinary excretion is markedly reduced, and fecal excretion increases. Results from excretion studies have been quite variable and have ranged from 28 to 88% of an administered dose for total 72-hour excretion.[5]

The exact mechanism by which pertechnetate concentrates in brain tumors is not known, but several factors are believed to play a role. The primary factor appears to involve a local disruption of the blood-brain barrier, with increased capillary permeability in the immediate vicinity of the lesion. Substances that cannot diffuse into normal brain tissue apparently cross the impaired barrier and pool in the pathologic tissues. It is also believed that the increased vascularity of the lesion contributes to the concentration of pertechnetate. It is theorized that pertechnetate binds to plasma proteins which serve to transport the radionuclide to the lesion. Generally, those lesions that demonstrate the greatest vascularity exhibit the greatest uptake of radionuclide.

GALLIUM-67

Physical Properties

Gallium-67 is a relatively new radionuclide that holds some promise as a tumor-localizing agent. It differs from previously described radionuclides in that it is produced in a cyclotron rather than in a nuclear reactor. In general, cyclotron-produced radionuclides are more expensive than radionuclides produced in a nuclear reactor. Gallium-67 is produced according to the nuclear transmutation reaction

$$^{67}Zn(p,n)^{67}GA$$

In actual practice, a zinc target is bombarded by a proton beam produced by the cyclotron. The nucleus of the zinc atom captures a proton and ejects a neutron, yielding the unstable ^{67}Ga nucleus. Gallium-67 decays by a complex mechanism known as electron capture. In general, this type of decay involves the capture of an orbital electron by the nucleus and the filling of the orbital vacancy by an electron from an outer shell. Characteristic γ rays are emitted in conjunction with the filling of each of the orbital vacancies. Several different energy γ rays are produced during the decay of ^{67}Ga, the most prominent of which are the 0.093 MeV, 0.184 MeV, 0.296 MeV, and 0.388 MeV energies. The T½ of ^{67}Ga is 78 hours. A simplified nuclear decay scheme is depicted below.

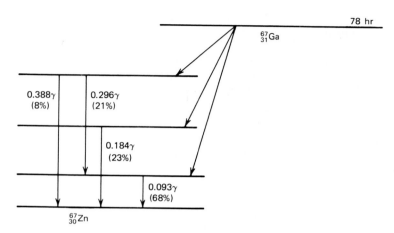

Chemical Properties

Gallium-67 is generally formulated as the citrate salt. Cyclotron targets are dissolved in sodium citrate, and diluted in physiological saline. Sterile, nonpyrogenic solutions of ^{67}Ga citrate are stable at room temperature.

Biological Properties

Gallium-67 distribution studies in humans have demonstrated high concentrations in the spleen, renal cortex, adrenals, and bone marrow, but tissue concentration values varied widely among the subjects studies.[6] Excretion has been shown to be both urinary and fecal.

The mechanism by which ^{67}Ga is concentrated in tumor tissue is not known, but it is speculated that Ga may bind to proteins that are taken up in rapidly proliferating cells.

IODINE-131

Physical Properties

Iodine-131 is one of the oldest and most widely used radionuclides in medicine. Prior to the widespread acceptance of ^{99m}Tc, radioiodine was employed in the large majority of nuclear medicine imaging procedures. Iodine-131 is produced in a nuclear reactor via the following neutron activation reaction:

$$^{130}Te \ (n,\gamma) \ ^{131}Te \xrightarrow{\beta^-} \ ^{131}I$$

In actual practice, a natural Te target is placed in the reactor neutron flux, where the

Te nucleus captures a neutron and expels a γ ray. The activated ^{131}Te produces ^{131}I as a result of β^- decay.

Iodine-131 decays by negatron emission producing several β^- particles and a number of γ rays. The primary β^- particles have a maximum energy of 0.33 MeV and 0.61 MeV, while the primary γ rays have energies of 0.36 MeV and 0.64 MeV. The T½ of ^{131}I is 8.1 days. A simplified nuclear decay scheme is depicted below.

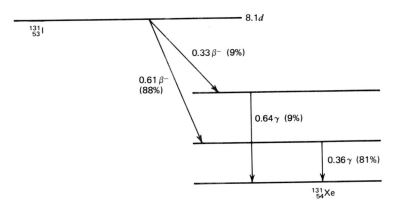

Chemical Properties

Iodine-131 is generally supplied as an aqueous solution of sodium iodide (NaI). It is used in this form for studies associated with the thyroid gland. Formulations of sodium iodide usually contain a reducing agent to keep the ^{131}I in the proper oxidation state, and parenteral formulations contain an appropriate preservative. In addition to use of the sodium iodide, ^{131}I has been tagged to a variety of compounds of medical interest for nuclear imaging and dynamic function studies.

Biological Properties

Iodine-131 is chemically identical to naturally occurring stable iodine (^{127}I) and is handled by the body in the same manner as stable iodine. Ingested iodine is rapidly absorbed, as iodide, from the intestinal tract and is removed from the bloodstream almost exclusively by the thyroid cells and the kidneys. The normal thyroid gland concentrates approximately 20% of the circulating iodide with each passage of blood through the gland. Iodide is concentrated to a lesser extent by the stomach and salivary glands. Excretion is almost entirely in the urine.

FUTURE APPLICATIONS

The radionuclides described above have contributed greatly to the application of nuclear medicine techniques to ophthalmology. Undoubtedly, certain of these radionuclides will be tagged to new and more specific compounds that will enhance their diagnostic utility. These advances, combined with advances in nuclear instrumentation, and the development of new radionuclides, promise to significantly broaden the impact of diagnostic nuclear medicine on ophthalmology in the years ahead.

REFERENCES

1. Thomas, C. I., Krohmer, J. S., and Storaasli, J. P.: Detection of Intraocular Tumors with Radioactive Phosphorus. *Arch. Ophthalmol.* **47**:276 (1952).

2. Reinhard, E. H. et al: Radioactive Phosphorus as a Therapeutic Agent. *J. Lab. Clin. Med.* **31**:107 (1946).

3. Harper, P. V. et al: Technetium-99m as a Biological Tracer. *J. Nuclear Med.* **3**:209 (1962).

4. Sodee, D. B.: The Study of Thyroid Physiology Utilizing Intravenous Sodium Pertechnetate. *J. Nuclear Med.* **7**:564 (1966).

5. Andros, G. et al: Pertechnetate-99m Localization in Man with Applications in Thyroid Scanning and the Study of Thyroid Physiology. *J. Clin. Endocrinol. Metab.* **25**:1067 (1965).

6. Nelson, W. et al: Distribution of Gallium in Human Tissues After Intravenous Administration. *J. Nuclear Med.* **13**:92 (1972).

Lesions of
the Uvea

CONTACT DETECTION
WITH RADIONUCLIDES

Problems and Improvements in the Diagnosis of Posterior Uveal Melanomas

Jerry A. Shields, M.D.
Senior Assistant Surgeon,
Retina Service,
Wills Eye Hospital,
Philadelphia, Pennsylvania

P. Robb McDonald, M.D.
Consultant, Retina Service,
Wills Eye Hospital;
Professor of Ophthalmology,
Thomas Jefferson University,
Philadelphia, Pennsylvania

Lov K. Sarin, M.D.
Attending Surgeon,
Retina Service,
Wills Eye Hospital;
Clinical Professor of Ophthalmology,
Thomas Jefferson University,
Philadelphia, Pennsylvania

It is well known that a variety of benign lesions in the ocular fundus may clinically simulate uveal malignant melanomas. In such cases, the ophthalmologist runs the risk of enucleating a useful eye containing a benign lesion. Judged by the number of reports in the ophthalmic literature, enucleations for such simulating lesions are not uncommon.[1-14]

Ferry, in an earlier report from the Armed Forces Institute of Pathology (AFIP), indicated the frequency of eyes enucleated for such simulating lesions.[1] In reviewing 7877 enucleations, he found 529 eyes that contained an ophthalmoscopically visible lesion diagnosed clinically as a posterior uveal melanoma. On histological examination, 100 of these eyes (19%), contained a lesion other than a malignant melanoma.

Ferry's study provoked considerable doubt that the percentage of erroneous diagnosis could be so high. Subsequently, other reports indicated a lower incidence of eyes enucleated for such simulating lesions.[2, 3] These reports, however, were from larger referral and teaching institutions where more tumors and suspected tumors are evaluated clinically. Ferry's study was probably more representative of the overall percentage in the United States.

Ferry speculated that with the advent of improved diagnostic techniques, the overall incidence of eyes enucleated for simulating lesions should decrease in subsequent years. To determine the validity of this prediction, Shields and Zimmerman updated Ferry's found that the incidence of eyes enucleated for simulating lesions was still 20%. Furthermore, a substantial number of these patients had not had the benefit of diagnostic procedures such as transillumination, fluorescein angiography, radioactive phosphorus uptake studies, ultrasound, or even indirect ophthalmoscopy.

Shields and McDonald recently reported the Wills Eye Hospital experience with so-called pseudomelanomas from 1962 through 1972. They demonstrated that the incidence of erroneous diagnosis was much less in a referral and teaching institution where patients with suspected uveal melanomas have the benefit of several ophthalmic consultations and evaluation with techniques now popular in the diagnosis of uveal melanomas.[15] This report updates their statistics through 1974.

METHODS

This study was conducted by reviewing all enucleations performed at Wills Eye Hospital during the 13-year period from 1962 through 1974. Except for the last 5 years, this study included the same years encompassed by the AFIP studies of Shields and Zimmerman.

Essentially the same criteria employed in the AFIP studies were utilized. We determined the number of eyes containing a visible fundus lesion that aroused enough suspicion to prompt enucleation. In some cases, the clinical diagnosis was malignant mel-

From the Oncology Unit, Retina Service, Wills Eye Hospital and Research Institute, Philadelphia, Pennsylvania. Supported in part by the Retina Research and Development Foundation, Philadelphia, Pennsylvania. Read before the 109th annual meeting of the American Ophthalmological Society, Hot Springs, Virginia, May 29, 1973. Presented by Dr. Lov K. Sarin at the 1st Symposium in Nuclear Ophthalmology, March 1975, Philadelphia, Pennsylvania.

anoma, whereas in other cases, the clinical impression was "possible melanoma" or "rule out melanoma." We then determined the incidence and type of enucleated eyes.

In order to study problems in diagnosis from another viewpoint, we listed the simulating lesions most frequently responsible for enucleation in the two series from the AFIP. We found the approximate number of such lesions seen on the Retina Service at Wills Eye Hospital since a unit of fundus photography and fluorescein angiography was established 8 years ago. We then determined the incidence of enucleation in our hospital for those lesions known to simulate posterior uveal melanoma.

RESULTS

During the 13-year period, 1610 enucleations were performed at Wills Eye Hospital. In 255 eyes (16%), the clinical diagnosis was melanoma or suspected melanoma. The media were opaque in 21 of these 255 eyes (8.2%). In 234 instances, the media were clear and the suspected lesion was visualized ophthalmoscopically. Of these 234 eyes, 7 were found on histological examination to harbor a simulating lesion rather than a malignant melanoma (3%) Table 1 illustrates the annual distribution of the simulating lesions during the 13-year period as well as the clinical and histopathologic diagnosis in each case. During the first 5 years of the study, there were 85 enucleations for suspected melanomas and 5 contained simulating lesions (6%). During the last 8 years (1967–1974), there were 149 enucleations and only 2 eyes contained simulating lesions (1.3%). Because these 7 eyes containing simulating lesions are the main concern of this report, further comment will be made on each case.

TABLE 1. DIAGNOSIS AND VISUAL ACUITY IN EYES ENUCLEATED FOR LESIONS SIMULATING MALIGNANT MELANOMA OF POSTERIOR UVEA[a]

Case	Year	Choroidal Diagnosis	Histopathologic Diagnosis	Visual Acuity
1	1963	Choroidal hemorrhage, rule out melanoma	Hemorrhagic retinal detachment	Light perception
2	1965	Intraocular tumor, possible melanoma	Hemorrhagic choroidal detachment	No light perception
3	1965	Malignant melanoma	Choroidal hemangioma	3/60
4	1965	Possible melanoma	Benign reactive lymphoid hyperplasia	6/6
5	1966	Malignant melanoma	Metastatic carcinoma to choroid from breast	6/12
6	1968	Amelanotic melanoma	Metastatic oat-cell carcinoma to choroid from lung	Count fingers at 1 ft
7	1971	Malignant melanoma	Metastatic carcinoma to choroid from gastrointestinal tract	Hand motions

[a] Wills Eye Hospital 1962–1974.

REPORT OF CASES

Case 1 (1963).   A 49-year-old white man had experienced poor vision in his left eye for about 1 year. About 3 days prior to admission, he noticed the sudden onset of sharp pain in the left eye. Visual acuity was 6/9 OD and light perception OS. Intraocular pressure was 13 mm Hg OD and 42 mm Hg OS (Schiotz). The patient had experienced myocardial infarctions in 1954 and 1962 and had been taking warfarin sodium (Coumadin) and digitalis for several years. Ocular examination revealed a complete bullous-shaped retinal detachment in the left eye. The clinical diagnosis was "subretinal hemorrhage left eye, possibly secondary to anticoagulants; rule out melanoma." Because a melanoma was not definitely ruled out, enucleation was performed. The histopathologic diagnosis was hemorrhagic retinal detachment (Fig. 1).

Case 2 (1965).   A 52-year-old white man had poor vision from the age of 14 when he experienced an episode of bilateral interstitial keratitis. Several years later, he had corneal transplants in both eyes. The right eye subsequently lost all vision and had had no light perception for 10 years. About 9 days prior to admission, he developed rather severe pain in the right eye. Ocular examination revealed a moderately hazy media due to corneal scarring in both eyes. In the right eye, a yellow-brown mass was observed nasally with a corresponding transillumination defect. Visual acuity was no light perception OD and 6/30 OS. The clinical diagnosis was probable intraocular neoplasm with phthisis bulbi, OD and old interstitial keratitis, OU. The histopathologic diagnosis was hemorrhagic choroidal detachment (Fig. 2).

Case 3 (1965).   A 73-year-old white man gave a history of painless progressive visual loss in his right eye for 6 months. Visual acuity was 3/60 OD and 6/6 OS. The intraocular pressures were normal OU. An elevated mass was noted superior to the macula with surrounding pigmentary dispersion. The clinical diagnosis was malignant melanoma and macular degeneration in the right eye. The histopathologic diagnosis was cavernous hemangioma of the choroid OD (Fig. 3).

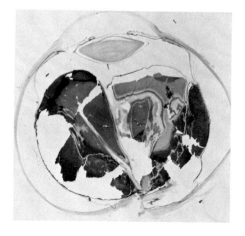

Fig. 1.   Section of enucleated left eye (case 1) showing total hemorrhagic detachment of retina (hematoxylin-eosin).

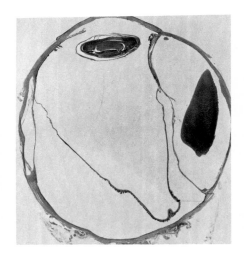

Fig. 2. Section of enucleated right eye (case 2) showing hemorrhagic detachment of choroid and ciliary body on nasal side. Retina is artifactiously detached on temporal side (hematoxylin-eosin).

Case 4 (1965). A 65-year-old white woman was seen by her ophthalmologist 2 weeks prior to admission because of floaters and flashes of light OS. Visual acuity was 6/6 OU and the intraocular pressures were normal. The diagnosis of retinal detachment was made by the patient's ophthalmologist and 15 Walker pins were inserted in the area of detachment. Several attempts to drain subretinal fluid were made, but no fluid could be obtained. Further consultations were obtained; the consensus was that this represented a solid detachment, and enucleation was advised.

Histopathologic examination revealed a diffuse infiltration of the choroid with lymphocytes on the nasal side and occasional plasma cells, probably a reactive lymphoid hyperplasia[16] (Fig. 4). Seven years later the patient was still alive and well.

Case 5 (1966). A 64-year-old white woman gave a 2-week history of persistent light flashes in her right eye. She had undergone a right mastectomy 3 years previously, apparently for breast carcinoma, but her present state of health was good. Visual acuity was 6/12 OD and 6/6 OS. Intraocular pressure was 15 mmHg OU (Schiotz). An elevated pigmented mass involving the ciliary body was seen superonasally OD. The clinical diagnosis was malignant melanoma of the ciliary body OD. The histopathologic diagnosis was metastatic adenocarcinoma from breast to the ciliary body with invasion of iris root and peripheral choroid (Fig. 5).

Case 6 (1968). A 56-year-old white woman noted painless progressive visual loss in her right eye for about 1 month. She had a sensation of looking through "yellow sunglasses." She was an obese lady with no physical complaints. X-ray films of the chest were interpreted as normal. Visual acuity was count fingers at 1 foot OD and 6/6 OS. Intraocular pressure was 13 mmHg OD and 16 mmHg OS (Schiotz). A nonpigmented moderately elevated mass was noted extending from the disc to the temporal equator OD. The clinical diagnosis was solid retinal detachment OD, possible malignant melanoma. The histopathologic diagnosis was metastatic oat-cell carcinoma to choroid from the lung (Fig. 6).

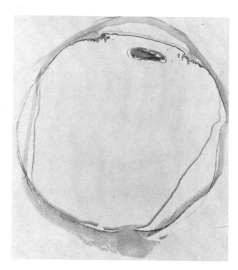

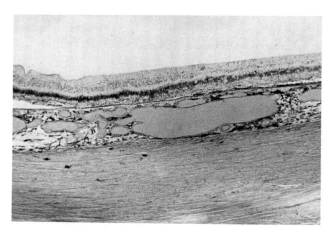

Fig. 3. Top: Enucleated right eye (case 3) showing diffuse placoid thickening of choroid temporally (hematoxylin-eosin). Bottom: Higher magnification showing large dilated cavernous blood vessels in choroid (hematoxylin-eosin ×32). Diagnosis was hemangioma of choroid.

Case 7 (1971). A 43-year-old white man had noted a progressive superonasal field defect in his left eye for 7 months. He had a history of a duodenal ulcer for many years, controlled by diet. An intraocular tumor had been noted in the left eye prior to admission. This was suspected to be a metastatic tumor, but a thorough medical evaluation including barium enema, x-ray films of the upper gastrointestinal tract, and liver biopsy had failed to reveal a primary lesion. Visual acuity was 6/6 OD and hand motions OS. Intraocular pressure was 17 mmHg OD and 16 mmHg OS (Schiotz). A large solid retinal detachment with a mottled yellow-brown surface was noted inferotemporally OS, extending to and involving the macula. Radioactive phosphorus (^{32}P) study revealed an uptake of 290% over the control eye. Because the medical evaluation failed to reveal a

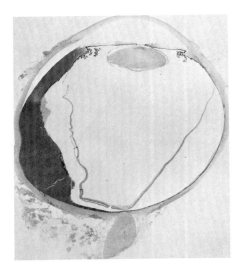

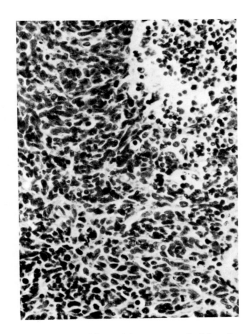

Fig. 4.   Left: Enucleated left eye (case 4) showing nasal thickening of uvea with overlying serous retinal detachment (hematoxylin-eosin). Right: Higher magnification showing numerous lymphocytes and occasional plasma cells (hematoxylin-eosin, ×320). Diagnosis was reactive lymphoid hyperplasia.

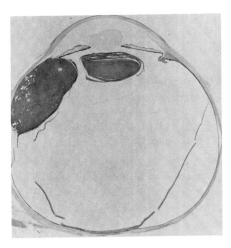

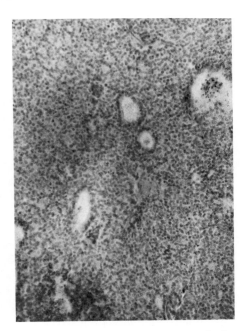

Fig. 5.   Left: Enucleated right eye (case 5) showing oval-shaped tumor involving peripheral uvea nasally (hematoxylin-eosin). Right: Higher magnification showing tumor cells around lumina (hematoxylin-eosin, ×128). Diagnosis was metastatic adenocarcinoma to choroid, presumably from breast.

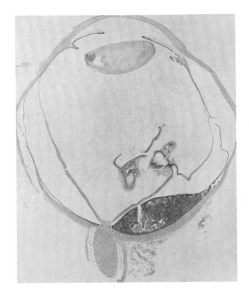 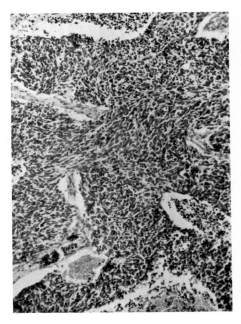

Fig. 6.   Left: Enucleated right eye (case 6) showing elevated choroidal mass temporally (hematoxylin-eosin). Right: Higher magnification showing densely arranged, oval-shaped cells (hematoxyline-eosin, ×128). Diagnosis was metastatic oat-cell carcinoma from lung to choroid.

primary neoplasm, the eye was enucleated as a suspected melanoma. The pathologic diagnosis was metastatic adenocarcinoma to the choroid, presumably from the gastrointestinal tract (Fig. 7).

It is important to note the visual acuity in the eyes that were enucleated for lesions simulating melanomas. These are shown in Table 1. It is significant that only two of the seven eyes had good vision (patients 4 and 5.) In the other five eyes, the visual acuity was less than 6/60.

It is noteworthy that in this series of 234 eyes containing a visible fundus lesion diagnosed clinically as a malignant melanoma or possible malignant melanoma, only 7 eyes, or 3%, were found on histological examination to harbor a lesion other than a melanoma. Five of the 7 eyes were enucleated during the first 5 years of the study, whereas only 2 of the 7 eyes were enucleated during the last 8 years.

During the last 8 years encompassed by this study, there was an active unit of fundus photography and fluorescein angiography, and patients with suspected fundus lesions were evaluated carefully by several observers. During these 8 years, there were 149 eyes with clear media that were enucleated for suspected uveal melanomas. Of these 149, only 2 eyes (1.3%) were found to harbor a simulating lesion. Both of these were metastatic tumors to the choroid, in eyes with poor vision, and both patients had been evaluated medically in search of a primary tumor (Table 1).

The percentage of erroneous diagnosis in this series was considerably lower than the reports from the AFIP[1, 4] and somewhat lower than other similar reports.[2 3] Several fac-

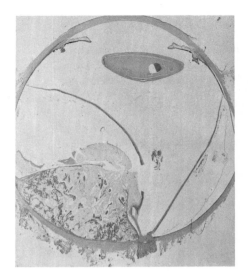
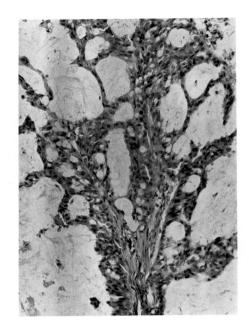

Fig. 7.   Left: Enucleated left eye (case 7) showing elevated mass in macular region with serous retinal detachment. Right: Higher magnification showing ribbons of tumor cells, occasional goblet cells, and mucin-folled spaces (hematoxylin-eosin, ×320). Diagnosis was metastatic adenocarcinoma from gastrointestinal tract to choroid.

tors probably played a role in reducing the percentage of erroneous diagnosis, especially during the last 8 years.

First is the apparent increase in the clinical awareness of such simulating lesions. This is largely due to a number of reports in the literature emphasizing the problems in differentiating such lesions from malignant melanomas.[1-14]

Another important factor is the increased use of the indirect ophthalmoscope. There is no question that with the bright illumination, the wider field of view, and stereopsis, one can better detect significant elevation of the retina, shifting fluid, and lesions underlying an elevated retina than with direct ophthalmoscopy.

Repeated fundus photography and fluorescein angiography are useful aids in the differential diagnosis of uveal melanomas.[17] During the last 6 years of this study, fluorescein angiography has been an integral part of the Retina Service, and repeated fundus photographs have been available to document any significant changes in suspected lesions. Although it is a useful procedure it is not diagnostic, as occasionally malignant melanomas will show no fluorescence[18] and benign nevi may sometimes fluoresce.[10]

It has long been recognized that transillumination is a useful diagnostic procedure in the differential diagnosis of uveal melanomas. This technique was routinely performed on the patients in this series and we believe that it is a useful diagnostic adjunct. In the case of posterior lesions, transillumination was usually performed on the operating table prior to enucleation.

In instances where the diagnosis of malignant melanoma is equivocal, several ophthalmological consultations are advisable prior to performing an enucleation. It is fortunate that in recent years suspected lesions seen in our institution were usually evaluated by several staff members of the Retina Service.

In recent years, the use of radioactive phosphorus uptake (^{32}P) has been revived as a diagnostic procedure in the evaluation of suspected fundus lesions.[19-22] Although this method has thus far not been helpful in differentiating a malignant melanoma from a metastatic choroidal neoplasm, it appears to be a useful adjunct in differentiating benign from malignant lesions. This procedure was utilized on more than 350 suspected cases during the last 4 years of this study, and the results have confirmed this impression. Thus far, however, it has not proved helpful in differentiating choroidal malignant melanomas from metastatic carcinomas.

Because of the low incidence of eyes enucleated for simulating lesions in this series, skeptics may raise two questions: first, whether we are actually seeing a significant number of lesions known to simulate uveal melanomas, and second, whether we may have lost to follow-up patients who actually had a uveal melanoma that was diagnosed as a simulating lesion.

In considering the first question, we listed the lesions most commonly confused with posterior uveal melanomas as derived from the two large studies from AFIP.[1, 4] We then reviewed our files to determine the number of such lesions seen either on consultation or for fluorescein angiography in the last 8 years of the study (1967–1974). Table 2 shows the approximate number of simulating lesions seen and the number of such lesions enucleated as suspected melanomas. During this 8-year period, the members of the Retina Service clinically evaluated more than 7600 lesions that may occasionally simulate posterior uveal melanomas.[1, 4] Only 2 of these 7600 were enucleated because a melanoma could not be ruled out. These were the two metastatic tumors to the choroid already mentioned (cases 6 and 7).

TABLE 2. LESIONS KNOWN TO SIMULATE POSTERIOR UVEAL MELANOMA[a]

Lesion	Approximate Number Seen	Number Enucleated as Suspected Melanomas
Rhegmatogenous retinal detachment	5730	0
Disciform macular degeneration	1330	0
Macular detachment (serous or hemorrhagic)	1070	0
Posterior uveitis	670	0
Choroidal nevus	530	0
Senile retinoschisis	530	0
Choroidal detachment	70	0
Metastatic carcinoma to choroid	70	2
Proliferation or hypertrophy of retinal pigment epithelium	70	0
Choroidal hemangioma	50	0
Melanocytoma of optic disc	15	0
Total	10,135	2

[a] Wills Eye Hospital 1962–1974.

The second question is more difficult to answer. To our knowledge no patients have been lost to follow-up who actually had a melanoma that was diagnosed on the Retina Service as something else. It is possible that some of the lesions that we diagnosed as benign, particularly the choroidal nevi, may have been malignant or may have subsequently become malignant. Attempts are routinely made, however, to obtain follow-up clinical evaluation, fundus photography, and fluorescein angiography in all such cases. In addition, ophthalmologists in this region would most likely inform us if they had seen a uveal melanoma that had not been properly diagnosed. In some instances, small pigmented fundus lesions were observed, but the eye was not enucleated until definite progression of the lesion was documented. To our knowledge, no patients have died as a result of this slight delay in enucleation, and we continue to advocate a conservative approach to equivocal fundus lesions.[10, 23] It has been pointed out that small malignant melanomas usually show more benign cytological features and that they usually have a better prognosis.[24] For this reason, a short period of careful observation seems justified. In one instance, the fluorescein angiograms done in our department were interpreted as a probable early melanoma, but enucleation was not advised. Enucleation was performed, however, in another hospital and the lesion proved to be a benign melanocytoma of the choroid. This case has been previously reported.[10]

It is important to recognize that the visual acuity was poor in five of the seven cases in this series. In the patient with no light perception enucleation was not objectionable and was perhaps even justified. In the study of Shields and Zimmerman, more than one-half of the eyes with simulating lesions had a vision of count fingers or less.[4]

Another important aspect of this study is that incidence of opaque media in eyes with malignant melanomas is considerably less than in previous studies. In most series of malignant melanomas, the incidence of opaque media has been about 21%.[4, 25, 26] In this study, the incidence of opaque media in the tumor-containing eyes was only 8.2%. It is likely that improved diagnostic techniques particularly indirect ophthalmoscopy have enabled smaller tumors to be detected and properly diagnosed before they become large enough to cause total retinal detachment and cataract. Despite our conservative approach to small equivocal lesions, we still advocate enucleation in most cases once the diagnosis of malignant melanoma is established.

We believe that the decreased incidence of eyes enucleated for lesions simulating uveal melanomas, especially during the last 8 years included in this study, has been largely a result of increased clinical awareness of such simulating lesions, as well as the use on the Retina Service of the diagnostic adjuncts mentioned above. The decision to enucleate an eye with a suspected lesion should not be made on the basis of any single test or procedure. Such a decision should be made on the basis of careful clinical observation in conjunction with the diagnostic adjuncts available.

SUMMARY

A total of 1610 consecutive enucleations performed at Wills Eye Hospital between 1962 and 1974 were reviewed. There were 234 eyes containing a visible fundus lesion which prompted enucleation because of a suspected malignant melanoma. On histological examination, 7 of these eyes (3%) were found to harbor a simulating lesion rather than a melanoma. During the last 8 years of this study, such simulating lesions were present in only 2 of 149 enucleated eyes, or 1.3%.

Several factors accounted for the decreased incidence of eyes enucleated for such simulating lesions. The most important factor was careful clinical observation, but other diagnostic adjuncts were useful in arriving at the diagnosis. In order to prevent unnecessary enucleations, it is recommended that every patient with a suspected fundus lesion be managed by the approach outlined.

REFERENCES

1. Ferry, A. P.: Lesions Mistaken for Malignant Melanoma of the Posterior Uvea. *Arch. Ophthalmol.* **72**:463 (1964).

2. Blodi, F. C., and Roy, P. E.: The Misdiagnosed Melanoma. *Can. J. Ophthalmol.* **2**:209 (1967).

3. Howard, G. M.: Erroneous Clinical Diagnosis of Retinoblastoma and Uveal Melanoma. *Trans. Am. Acad. Ophthalmol. Oto.* **73**:199 (1969).

4. Shields, J. A., and Zimmerman, L. E.: Lesions Simulating Malignant Melanoma of the Posterior Uvea. *Arch. Ophthalmol.* **89**:466 (1973).

5. Zimmerman, L. E.: Problems in the Diagnosis of Malignant Melanoma of the Choroid and Ciliary Body. The Arthur J. Bedell Lecture, 1972. *Am. J. Ophthalmol.* **75**:917 (1973).

6. Zimmerman, L. E.: Symposium: Macular Diseases, Macular Lesions Mistaken for Malignant Melanoma of the Choroid. *Trans. Am. Acad. Ophthalmol. Oto.* **69**:623 (1965).

7. Rones, B., and Zimmerman, L. E.: An Unusual Choroidal Hemorrhage Simulating a Malignant Melanoma. *Arch. Ophthalmol.* **70**:30 (1963).

8. Ferry, A. P.: Macular Detachment Associated with Congenital Pit of the Optic Nervehead. *Arch. Ophthalmol.* **70**:346 (1963).

9. Gordon, E.: Nevus of the Choroid and Pars Plana. *Surv. Ophthalmol.* **3**:507 (1963).

10. Shields, J. A., and Font, R. L.: Melanocytoma of the Choroid Clinically Simulating a Malignant Melanoma. *Arch. Ophthalmol.* **87**:396 (1972).

11. Tredici, T. J., and Fenton, R. H.: Hematoma Beneath the Retinal Pigment Epithelium: Report of a Case Mistaken Clinically for a Malignant Melanoma of the Choroid. *Arch. Ophthalmol.* **72**:796 (1964).

12. Vogel, M., Zimmerman, L. E., and Gass, J. D. M.: Proliferation of the Juxtapapillary Retinal Pigment Epithelium Simulating a Malignant Melanoma. *Doc. Ophthalmol.* **4**:469 (1969).

13. Berkow, J. W., and Font, R. L.: Disciform Macular Degeneration with Subpigment Epithelial Hematoma. *Arch. Ophthalmol.* **82**:51 (1969).

14. Zimmerman, L. E., and Spencer, W. H.: The Pathologic Anatomy of Retinoschisis with a Report of Two Cases Diagnosed Clinically as Malignant Melanoma. *Arch. Ophthalmol.* **63**:10 (1960).

15. Shields, J. A., and McDonald, P. Robb: Improvements in the Diagnosis of Posterior Uveal Melanomas. *Tran. Am. Ophthalmol. Soc.* **71**:193 (1973), *Arch. Ophthalmol.* **91**:259 (1974).

16. Ryan, S. J., Zimmerman, L. E., and King, S. M.: Reactive Lymphoid Hyperplasia: An Unusual Form of Intraocular Pseudotumor. *Tran. Am. Acad. Ophthalmol. Oto.* **76**:652 (1972).

17. Norton, E. et al: Fluorescein Fundus Photography: An Aid in the Diagnosis of Posterior Ocular Lesions. *Trans. Am. Acad. Ophthalmol. Oto.* **68**:755 (1964).

18. Shields, J. A., Annesley, W. H., and Totino, J. A.: Nonfluorescent Malignant Melanoma of the Choroid Diagnosed with the Radioactive Phosphorus Uptake Test. *Am. J. Ophthalmol.* **79**:634 (1975).

19. Hagler, W. S., Jarrett, W. H. II, and Humphrey, W. T.: The Radioactive Phosphorus Uptake Test in the Diagnosis of Uveal Melanoma. *Arch. Ophthalmol.* **83**:548 (1970).

20. Shields, J. A., Sarin, L. K., Federman, J. L. Mensheha-Manhart, O., and Carmichael, P. L.: Surgical Approach to the ^{32}P Test for Posterior Uveal Melanomas. *Ophthalmol. Surg.* **5**:13 (1974).

21. Shields, J. A., Hagler, W. S., Federman, J. L., Jarrett, W. H., and Carmichael, P. L: The Significance of the ^{32}P Test in the Diagnosis of Posterior Uveal Melanomas. *Trans. Am. Acad. Ophthalmol. Oto.* **79**:297 (1975).

22. Shields, J. A., Carmichael, P. L., Leonard, B. C., Federman, J. L., and Sarin, L. K.: The Accuracy of the ^{32}P Test for Ocular Melanomas. An Analysis of 350 cases. Presented at AMA Section on Ophthalmology Meeting June, 1975 (submitted for publication).

23. Shields, J. A., Green, W. R., and McDonald, P. R.: Uveal Pseudomelanoma due to Post-traumatic Pigmentary Migration. *Arch. Ophthalmol.* **89**:519 (1973).

24. Flocks, M., Gerende, J. H., and Zimmerman, L. E.: The Size and Shape of Malignant Melanomas of the Choroid and Ciliary Body in Relation to the Prognosis and Cystologic Characteristics: A Statistical Study of 210 Tumors. *Trans. Am. Acad. Ophthalmol. Oto.* **59**:740 (1955).

25. Makley, T. A., and Teed, R. W.: Unsuspected Intraocular Malignant Melanomas. *Arch. Ophthalmol.* **60**:475 (1958).

26. Jensen, O. A.: Malignant Melanomas of the Uvea in Denmark 1943–1952: A Clinical, Histopathological, and Prognostic Study. *Acta Ophthalmol.* (Suppl.) **75**:1–220 (1963).

Contact Detection with Radionuclides—The Instruments

C. Craig Harris, M.S.
Associate Professor of Radiology,
Division of Nuclear Medicine,
Department of Radiology,
Duke University Medical Center,
Durham, North Carolina

The specialized characteristics of instruments for detection of radiation from radionuclides are dictated in part by the physical configuration encountered and in part by the properties of the radiations encountered. In detecting radioactivity in the orbit, the physical configuration demands the capability for a high degree of localization. This requires either a detector with a very high-resolution focused collimator (for gamma or x-ray photons) or a very small detector that may be placed close to a source of beta particles.

The former has not achieved a high state of development chiefly because of the lack of widespread use of gamma-emitting radionuclides in studies of small organs (e.g., eye and thyroid). The use of low-energy gamma or x-ray emitters such as Iodine-125 in radiopharmaceuticals for these organs would permit the use of a small, high-resolution focused scintillation probe simply because it would require only a thin crystal and a small amount of material in the focused collimator. (A gamma eye probe with a nonfocused, flat-field collimator for use with ^{125}I compounds has recently become commercially available.*)

Sources of beta particles are best studied with a small detector in contact, because the intensity of beta radiation falls off rapidly with distance from the source. Hence, counting rates and therefore localizing ability are maximum with a detector in contact with, or as close as possible to, the source.

A small contact detector for beta particles has been available for many years. Its availability has been based chiefly on the use of phosphorus-32 in studies of intraocular tumors. The range of ^{32}P beta particles in tissue is sufficiently great that over half can penetrate 2 mm of tissue;[1] those of intraocular origin can therefore be detected externally.

The first contact detectors developed were small specialized Geiger-Müller (G-M) detectors,[2] which underwent later improvements.[3] More recently, these have been joined by semiconductor detectors in similar physical forms.[4] Because there are two types available and because some knowledge of the instrumental considerations of contact detection is useful in any event, this discussion is offered.

GEIGER-MÜLLER DETECTORS AND COUNTING SYSTEMS

Geiger-Müller (G-M) detectors were chosen for development into small specialized forms, probably because at the time the G-M detector was more commonly used than any other and because it employed the simplest associated electronic circuits. The simplicity derives from the fact that a G-M detector is operated so that the interaction of ionizing radiation results in rapid ionization of virtually all the gas in the device.[5] The result is a large output voltage pulse, the size of which is nearly the same from one event to another, and which requires little, if any, amplification for recording by a scaler or ratemeter.

Actual G-M Detector Probes and Systems

Figure 1, taken from commercial literature,** shows several forms of currently available G-M detector probes and provides some idea of their small size. The two probes at the

* Technical Associates, 7051 Eton Avenue, Canoga Park, California 91303.
** EON Corporation, 175 Pearl Street, Brooklyn, New York 11201.

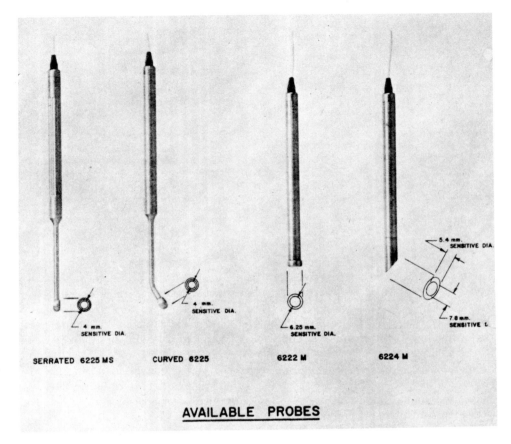

AVAILABLE PROBES

Fig. 1. Various G-M ocular detectors, taken from an illustration in commercial literature. The two detector probes at left are in most common use.

left of the illustration are designed to pass posteriorly to the orbit. Figure 2 shows the actual detectors in more detail. The modern form, with a stainless steel foil (0.0002 in. thick) entrance window, and rim serrations is shown at lower right (5 o'clock position). An older form (as originally designed) is shown with its nearly transparent mica window at lower left (8 o'clock position). The probe at the extreme right is generally limited to use in the anterior aspects of the orbit.

A complete G-M detector system, including a high voltage supply, a scaler, a count rate meter, an aural count indicator ("chirper"), and an indicating timer, is shown in Figure 3.* A foot switch initiates a timed counting interval; the timer terminates the interval with both time and count displayed. The "chirper" operates continuously and is very useful in locating points of maximum activity. Also shown is an important accessory, a plate with clips and cleats on which the probe and its cable are mounted for gas sterilization. Not shown but available and equally important is a standard source apparatus into which the probe can be inserted and clamped for calibration and checking.

* EON Corporation.

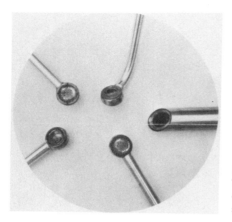

Fig. 2. A close-up view of several G-M ocular detectors. The probes nearest top and bottom are in current use. The entrance window of these two detectors is 0.0002-in. thick stainless steel foil.

Operating Considerations

The lack of strong dependence of observed counting rate on applied high voltage, or the typical "plateau" in G-M detector operation, provides a considerable operating convenience. Very few G-M detectors, however, have an ideal "plateau." Even large G-M detectors of nearly optimum construction show some slight increase of counting rate above the "knee" of the counting rate curve. In other words, counting rate is in reality at least slightly dependent on applied high voltage.

Small ocular G-M probes exhibit a considerably poorer plateau, requiring that they be set to a high voltage that gives a standard response to a long-lived source. Once set, operation is stable for several hours. A procedure that is usually satisfactory is to start with minimum high voltage and increase it until counts from a standard source just begin. Operation at 50–100 V higher than the threshold setting usually is stable and safe. Excessive high voltage will damage and may even destroy the counter.

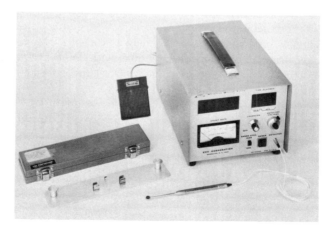

Fig. 3. A complete, commercially available G-M ocular probe system. The system includes a high voltage supply, a scaler, a ratemeter, an indicating timer, an audible count indicator, and a foot switch to initiate a counting period.

A G-M detector in which the threshold value of high voltage slowly increases (over an hour or so) by as much as 50–100 V is in an unsuitable condition. It can be trusted only over short periods of time, and only then by constant checking on a standard source.

While the entrance window of the modern G-M ocular detector (0.0002 in. stainless steel) is much more durable than the previous mica window,[3] it can be damaged by rough handling. The serrated peripheral face (Fig. 2) of the modern detector minimizes slippage over the scleral surface.

Gas sterilization causes no damage to the detector probe and cable itself but may cause tarnishing of the cable connector, resulting in poor contact and erratic operation. This tarnishing may be minimized by plugging the cable connector into an unmounted mating chassis connector, which serves as a cover during sterilization. This operational factor also applies to semiconductor probes.

SEMICONDUCTOR DETECTORS AND SYSTEMS

The semiconductor detector, particularly the lithium-drifted silicon (SiLi) detector, is very well suited for fabrication into a small ocular contact detector. In fact, modern semiconductor ocular detectors are quite similar in appearance to the earlier developed G-M probe.

Figure 4 shows a probe assembly with two detachable detector units, the disc-shaped one being intended for ocular use.* The handle contains the necessary preamplifier, which supplies the relatively low operating voltage (24 volts) to the detector. Different forms of detector units are shown in Fig. 5.* Sizes are comparable with G-M detectors (larger units in Fig. 5) but a smaller (2 mm active diameter) one also is shown in Figure 6.* A similar system using the same detector is shown in Figure 7.**

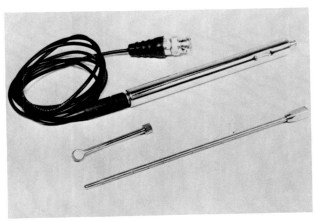

Fig. 4. A commercially available pair of semiconductor detectors with their common preamplifier-handle-cable combination.

---

* Probes and counting system as marketed by Technical Associates, Canoga Park, California. Standard probe and counting system also available from Nuclear Associates, 35 Urban Avenue, Westbury, New York 11590. Detectors are manufactured by Solid State Radiations, Inc., 2261 South Carmelina Avenue, Los Angeles, California 90064.
** Tennelec, Inc., 601 Turnpike, Oak Ridge, Tennessee 37830.

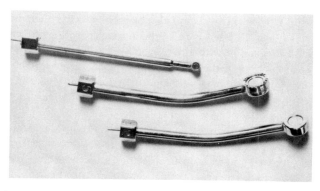

Fig. 5. Additional detector units for the probe assembly of Fig. 4. Sizes are comparable with G-M detectors, these being slightly larger.

Another type of semiconductor detector, called a "silicon avalanche detector,"[6] is the solid-state analog of gas proportional counters. These devices have low noise and high detection sensitivity owing to internal amplification and a thin entrance window; they operate at very high voltages, 1000–2000 V. They are available commercially† but are not yet in widespread use. Except for the necessary high voltage supply, the electronic instruments used for lithium-drifted silicon detectors are suitable for use with silicon avalanche detectors.

Operating Considerations

While the "background" count from a G-M detector is usually due only to actual detected radiation, the SiLi detector internally generates noise pulses to which the external circuits can respond. Figure 8 shows pulse height spectra resulting from detection of ^{32}P beta particles by a SiLi detector of the type shown in Fig. 5. The spectra are on semi-logarithmic (upper) and linear (lower) coordinates. The letters A and B denote response

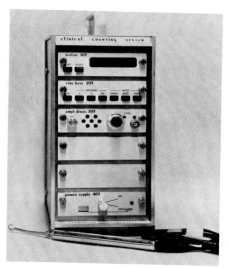

Fig. 6. A commercially available complete semiconductor ocular probe and counting system. The control marked "LEVEL" is the control referred to in the text as a "threshold control."

† The General Electric Company, Philadelphia, Pennsylvania.

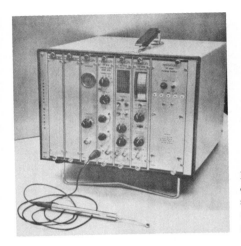

Fig. 7. A commercially available semiconductor ocular probe and counting system. The detector is the same as in Fig. 6, while the remainder of the system is assembled from AEC-NIM (Atomic Energy Commission-Nuclear Instrument Module) units.

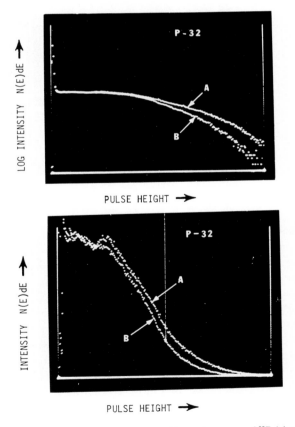

Fig. 8. Pulse height spectra from a SiLi ocular detector with a point source of ^{32}P (*a*) and a 1 cc liquid source of ^{32}P (*b*), on semilogarithmic coordinates (upper) and on linear coordinates (lower). Note the very high noise level at low pulse height (upper left in upper spectra).

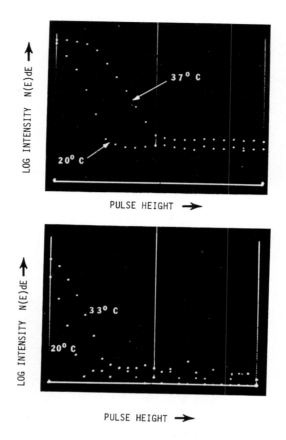

Fig. 9. Expanded pulse height spectra from a SiLi ocular detector with a ^{32}P source (upper) and with background only (lower) at two probe temperatures. Low-energy-equivalent noise increases considerably with probe temperature.

to point and volume sources, respectively. A high intensity of very small pulses may be seen at the upper left of the log spectrum. These pulses are always present; counts providing the remainder of the spectra vanish when the source is removed. In the electronics of the system, a threshold discriminator is provided to reject these noise pulses and pass those due to detection of beta particles.

Unfortunately, the noise level increases with temperature, and a threshold set to pass a maximum of detection pulses (just above the noise) at a low temperature would be exceeded by noise pulses at a higher temperature. Figure 9 shows pulse height spectra with a source present (upper) and with only background radiation (lower). The scale is such that only the pulse heights at the left margin of the spectra of Fig. 8 are shown. The increased noise at operating temperatures at slightly below body levels is readily evident. This can be a definite problem if the threshold is set at the edge of the noise spectrum with the probe at room temperature (20°–22° C); when the ophthalmologic surgeon's hand (and the patient's eye) warm the probe, it can begin responding to the noise. This can shatter the confidence of all present and send the instrument away for needless repair.

In setting the threshold at our institution, we warm the probe (with water) to around 37°–40° C. This reduces sensitivity but prevents noise problems due to the shifting threshold. Ideally, the probe should be operating as long as possible before use. Additionally, dipping it in warm sterile saline not only keeps it near body temperature but also cleanses it between uses. Gas sterilization is harmless to the SiLi probe and cable, but as with the G-M probe, connector tarnishing must be prevented.

WHICH IS BETTER, G-M OR SEMICONDUCTOR?

Larose and colleagues, with the cooperation of other investigators and detector developers, performed some comparisons of G-M, silicon surface-barrier, diffused junction, lithium-drifted, and avalanche detectors.[7] This comparison cites comparable performance among all the silicon devices except the avalanche detector, which is more sensitive and more temperature dependent. The avalanche detector presented some problems, chiefly due to its developmental nature. Also related is a disenchantment with the fragility and lack of stability of G-M detectors.

At Duke University Medical Center, we began performance of ^{32}P eye tumor identification studies with the G-M system shown in Fig. 3. We found it stable and reliable, though one of the two detectors developed a shifting plateau and had to be replaced. In particular, the operational properties of the system made it convenient to use.

Later we acquired a silicon detector (Fig. 4), put together a system similar to that in Fig. 7, and used both instruments on a few patients with identical results in terms of tumor-to-control ratio. We discovered the thermal sensitivity of the semiconductor probe. Counting rates were somewhat higher (10 to 40%) with the semiconductor probe, even with the loss of sensitivity from an elevated threshold.

We concluded that both systems were quite satisfactory, the differences consisting mostly of operational detail. Our silicon probes do not have serrated rims, but with care their use is satisfactory; current probes do have serrated edges. We did not retain the G-M system, which was present for procedure evaluation, solely because of capital equipment fund limitations; the silicon detector systems used modular equipment already on hand. The G-M system's performance was satisfactory and convenient; the same can be said for the semiconductor system.

It is our opinion that the differences in systems and detector types probably are less than the differences between proper and improper performance of the procedure. Larose[7] states: "The ^{32}P eye-tumor identification test is a useful diagnostic tool if performed correctly. It is mandatory that the detector be placed directly over the lesion or else false negative tests will nullify its usefulness." While our limited instrument comparison did not yield impressions of detector quality quite the same as those formed by the far more complete study of Larose, Hagler, and Jarrett, we nevertheless concur most vigorously with their insistence in placing the counter over the lesion. Both G-M and semiconductor probes have the physical attributes to be placed over the lesion, and both seem to perform correctly when properly placed and the system is properly adjusted. By the same reasoning, neither type can produce satisfactory results if placed poorly and handled improperly.

REFERENCES

1. Carmichael, P. L., Holst, G. G., Federman, J. L., and Shields, J. A.: The Present Status of the ^{32}P Test in Ophthalmology. In Croll, M. N., Brady, L. W., Honda, T., and Wallner, R. J., Eds., *New Techniques in Tumor Localization and Radioimmunoassay,* John Wiley, New York, 1974.

2. Thomas, C. I., Bovington, M. S., and MacIntyre, W. J.: Experimental Investigations on Uptake of Radioactive Phosphorus in Ocular Tumors. *Arch. Ophthalmol.* (Chicago) **61**:464 (1959).

3. Ruiz, R. S.: New Radioactivity Detection Probe and Scaler for Phosphorus-32 Testing of Ocular Lesions. *Trans. Am. Acad. Ophthalmol. Otolaryn.* Mar.-Apr. (1972).

4. Friedland, S. S., Benary, V., Ewins, J. H., and Katzenstein, H. S.: In Vivo Silicon Detectors, in Vivo Preamplifiers and Their Applications. *IEEE Trans. Nuclear Sci.* **NS-19** (June 1952).

5. Robinson, C. V.: Geiger-Müller and Proportional Counters. In Hine, G. J., (Ed., *Instrumentation in Nuclear Medicine,* Academic Press, New York, 1967.

6. Huth, G. C., and Moldofsky, P. J.: Avalanche Semiconductor Detectors. In Hoffer, P. B., Beck, R. N., and Gottschalk, A., Eds., *Semiconductor Detectors in The Future of Nuclear Medicine,* Society of Nuclear Medicine, Inc., New York, 1971, Chapter 6.

7. Larose, J. H.: Semiconductor Detectors for Eye-Tumor Diagnosis. In Hoffer, P. B., Beck, R. N., and Gottschalk, A., Eds., *Semiconductor Detectors in the Future of Nuclear Medicine.* Society of Nuclear Medicine, Inc., New York, 1971, Chapter 13.

Ten Years' Experience with Radioactive Phosphorus Uptake Test in the Diagnosis of Uveal Malignancy

William H. Jarrett II, M.D.
Clinical Associate Professor of Ophthalmology,
Medical School of Georgia,
Augusta, Georgia

The diagnosis and management of tumors of the uveal tract are two of the most challenging and difficult tasks confronting the ophthalmologist. Two major forms of malignant tumors occur in the uvea: primary malignant melanoma of the uvea and neoplasms metastatic to the uvea from a primary site elsewhere in the body. However, a variety of nonneoplastic lesions may also involve the uveal tract and mimic a potentially lethal tumor. The problem is to differentiate the former from the latter because proper management depends on accurate and precise diagnosis.

A number of recent studies in the ophthalmic literature attest to the difficulties encountered in making this differential diagnosis.[1-4] The study by Ferry in 1964, updated by Shields and Zimmerman in 1973, indicates that approximately one eye in five removed with the clinical diagnosis of malignant melanoma does not, in fact, contain a melanoma. Eyes containing benign lesions such as choroidal hemangioma, choroidal nevus, serous or hemorrhagic detachment of the retinal pigment epithelium, or melanocytoma of the optic nerve head have been unnecessarily removed. And this, of course, is only one side of the problem viewed from the standpoint of the ocular pathologist examining material submitted to his laboratory. What about those eyes harboring malignancies that go undiagnosed, but which should be removed?[5, 6] How many eyes, for example, undergo scleral buckling surgery for retinal detachment, when, in fact, the detachment is not a rhegmatogenous one but is secondary to a choroidal tumor?[7, 8] A malignant tumor of the uveal tract is a potentially lethal disease; even the "benign" spindle A melanoma carries a significant 5-year mortality rate. Thus, it behooves us as clinicians to separate the benign from the malignant tumors and treat the patient accordingly.

How do we go about making this differentiation clinically? There is no question that a careful examination of the ocular fundus, utilizing stereoscopic binocular indirect ophthalmoscopy, slit lamp fundus contact lens, and fluorescein angiography will lead to the correct diagnosis in the vast majority of cases, probably 90% or better. But nonetheless, there remain a number of cases where the clinical diagnosis is uncertain. Biopsy of the lesion in the wall of the eye is not recommended, because (1) the procedure itself is hazardous and might result in loss of useful vision, and (2) if the lesion being biopsied is a neoplasm, the procedure might spread the tumor into the orbit.

In our hands the most useful tool for making the distinction between a benign and malignant lesion of the choroid or ciliary body is the radioactive phosphorus ^{32}P uptake test. I have deliberately excluded iris lesions from the discussion, because I have not found the ^{32}P test useful in identifying iris melanomas. A combination of factors accounts for this, including (1) the relatively small mass of iris lesions, and (2) the corneal thickness and the depth of the anterior chamber, which separate the iris lesion from the counting probe. I no longer perform ^{32}P testing in patients with iris lesions.

RADIOPHOSPHORUS

Radiophosphorus is a colorless, odorless liquid isotope of phosphorus with a half-life of 14 days. It emits only beta particles. Actively metabolizing cells have been shown to incorporate phosphorus in their metabolic cycle, and thus with the passage of time ^{32}P will accumulate in such tissue. By utilizing the radioactive isotope of phosphorus, the clinician is afforded a means of measuring this accumulation and comparing it with other, presumably normal, tissue. A high concentration of ^{32}P in a tissue often denotes the presence of a malignancy, but sites such as healing surgical wounds, with granulation tissue, can also concentrate [32]P. Thomas[9] first described the use of ^{32}P in detecting ocular tumors, and Dunphy,[10] Carmichael,[11]. Leopold,[12] and others have contributed to our knowledge of this diagnostic modality.

CLINICAL EXPERIENCE

Since 1965, Hagler and I[13, 14] have been using the ^{32}P test routinely in our evaluation of patients presenting with masses of the uveal tract. Initially, the test was performed as an ancillary adjunct in eyes that were to be enucleated anyway with a clinical diagnosis of malignant melanoma. It soon became apparent, however, that the test was uniformly positive in eyes that were shown pathologically to contain a malignancy. From these beginnings, we moved to utilize the ^{32}P test in cases where the diagnosis was not so obvious clinically, and we are now at the point where we consider it the single most helpful diagnostic test available in the differential diagnosis of a uveal mass. In our hands, a positive ^{32}P test is strong evidence pointing to the diagnosis of an ocular neoplasm. Likewise, a negative ^{32}P test is highly significant and good evidence against the existence of an ocular malignancy.

Certain refinements in the technique of performing the test have proved invaluable, especially for posteriorly placed lesions. We have utilized a conjunctival incision, mobilization of the globe with traction sutures under the muscles, and accurate localization of the tumor with indirect ophthalmoscopy, marking the sclera with diathermy so as to locate on the surface of the globe the exact position of the underlying choroidal tumor. The counting probe can then be positioned directly over the lesion and readings taken. Accurate and precise localization of the tumor cannot be stressed too strongly because radioactive phosphorus is a beta emitter, and beta particles travel only a few millimeters in tissue. If the probe is not directly over the lesion, falsely low (false-negative) readings may occur. We think that this probably occurred with small, posteriorly placed lesions when the conjunctiva was not incised in the early phase of ^{32}P testing, and was one reason the test fell into disrepute.

The modification in technique just described is not original with us. As fellows on the Retinal Service at the Massachusetts Eye and Ear Infirmary, we observed this technique being utilized by Dr. Charles Schepens and his associates in similar cases.

Before describing our clinical experiences with ^{32}P testing, let me outline our evaluation of a patient presenting with a choroidal tumor mass. A complete ophthalmic and medical history is taken with particular reference to any history of neoplasm elsewhere in the body. Such a patient receives a thorough eye examination, and the suspicious lesion is studied with indirect ophthalmoscopy, slit lamp contact lens examination, transillumination, contact B-scan ultrasonography, and fluorescein angiography. At this stage, we consider the ^{32}P test. We do not do the test, for instance, on lesions we think are nevi clinically, or on post operative choroidal detachments. This involves making a clinical judgment on the basis of what we see in the eye, and quite obviously this judgment is not infallible.

In the majority of cases of uveal masses, ^{32}P testing is done. The patient is admitted to the hospital, where a thorough medical evaluation is performed by a qualified internist who knows that a tumor is suspected and who knows to look for a primary site of neoplasm or evidence of distant metastases. Complete blood studies, including SMA 12, urinalysis, and chest x-ray are routinely done. We do not request more extensive procedures such as GI series, barium enema, or IVP as part of a routine work-up, since these have proved to be nonproductive in most patients. However, if the history or physical findings indicate, then these tests are carried out.

The ^{32}P is administered intravenously by the Department of Nuclear Medicine. This material can only be obtained by a practitioner of nuclear medicine who is licensed to use that particular isotope. The cooperation of the Department of Nuclear Medicine has been of utmost importance and invaluable to us in putting together this series of cases.

Forty-eight hours after the ^{32}P injection, the readings are made in the operating room. After localizing the lesion as described earlier, several readings are taken over the lesion, and at least three readings are taken over each of the other three "control" quadrants in the same eye. We do not use the fellow eye to get our "control" readings. These results are then averaged and utilized in the formula

$$\frac{C_L - C_N}{C_N} \times 100 = {}^{32}\text{P uptake}$$

where C_L = counts over lesion, and C_N = counts over the normal quadrants.

We consider a 65% ^{32}P uptake, or greater, a positive test. However, in the vast majority of patients with ocular malignancies, the ^{32}P is well over 100% and frequently is in the range of 200–300%. We have had experience with both the solid-state and the EON instruments and feel that both give satisfactory results in the clinical setting.

From January 1, 1965, through December 31, 1974, we have performed a total of 231 ^{32}P tests. The results are as follows:

Total ^{32}P Tests

 A. Positive Tests 185
   (False-positive: 1)
 B. Negative Tests 46
   (No known false-negative test)

Positive ^{32}P Test. A positive ^{32}P test resulted in 185 cases. Only one of these is known known to be a false-positive test. This involved a lesion of the peripheral choroid in a 34-year-old Negro male in which the ^{32}P test was 122% positive. The eye was removed and the lesion was diagnosed histologically as benign adenoma of the retinal pigment epithelium.

Of the remaining 184 cases, the histopathologic diagnosis is known in 161 cases, and in every single case the lesion was a neoplasm. In 23 instances, we do not know the histopathology, either because the eye was not removed for one reason or another or because we have not been able to obtain the necessary information. In view of these statistics, we feel justified in stating that a positive ^{32}P test is very strong evidence indeed for the presence of an ocular malignancy.

As stressed earlier, most of the 156 cases of melanoma were easily diagnosable clinically, and the positive ^{32}P readings were not unexpected. Thus, one of the questions that we are frequently asked is, How often has the ^{32}P test been *really* useful and told you something you do not already know? The answer to this question is, not often, but it does happen. The following cases should illustrate this point.

Case 1. Choroidal melanoma in a 14-year-old white female, correctly diagnosed with ^{32}P testing.

This 14-year-old white female presented with a choroidal mass lesion in the left eye.

The vision in the eye was reduced to 20/50. The lesion was slightly elevated, moderately pigmented, and the superior edge of the lesion involved the macula. A ^{32}P test done at this time was positive, but because of the patient's age she was referred to another center for consultation. The consultant felt very strongly that the lesion was a benign disturbance of the retinal pigment epithelium and advised against enucleation. Six months later the lesion had enlarged in size and a serous retinal detachment had appeared. The ^{32}P test was repeated and again markedly positive. The globe was removed, and the lesion was a spindle B melanoma of the choroid.

Case 2. Malignant melanoma diagnosed by ^{32}P testing in a case being followed with a clinical diagnosis of choroidal hemangioma.

A 32-year-old white female was referred with a choroidal tumor mass in the right eye. This mass had first been discovered 2 years earlier and was associated with a serous secondary retinal detachment. The diagnosis of a malignant melanoma was entertained and enucleation was scheduled. However, in the operating room, it was noted that the lesion in question blanched upon compression and that no transillumination defect was visible. These two factors gave the surgeon pause; enucleation was cancelled, and the patient was referred for further consultation. Several experienced consultants saw the patient and diagnosed hemangioma of the choroid, and the patient was treated with photocoagulation and followed. However, in that time the lesion grew and the serous detachment did not disappear despite the photocoagulation treatment. When the ^{32}P test was performed, the test was markedly positive (142%) and the eye was enucleated. Histopathologically, this lesion proved to be a spindle B melanoma of the choroid.

The foregoing are instances where the ^{32}P test has been helpful to us in establishing the correct diagnosis in difficult and challenging cases where there was a legitimate difference of opinion between experienced and expert clinicians. It thus illustrates the diagnostic potential of this modality.

METASTATIC TUMORS

In five instances, we have enucleated eyes harboring choroidal tumor masses that were thought to be malignant melanomas clinically, only to learn from histopathologic examination that the lesion was a carcinoma metastatic to the choroid. In each of these cases, the patient was not known to have a tumor elsewhere, and the ocular metastasis was the first sign of the disease. These lesions were pigmented collar button tumors, indicating extension through Bruch's membrane, and fluoresced with intravenous fluorescein. All of these characteristics point toward a diagnosis of malignant melanoma. In addition, no primary tumor had been discovered in the preoperative medical evaluation. Indeed, in several instances, a primary tumor could not be found despite very intensive medical evaluation once the lesion had been found to be a metastatic tumor. In these cases, it was many months before the primary tumor, usually a bronchogenic carcinoma became manifest.

NEGATIVE ^{32}P TEST

In our series of cases, a total of 46 negative ^{32}P tests have been encountered. In none of these cases is histopathologic material available, and thus we cannot categorically state that the lesion in question is, in fact, benign. The clinical diagnoses made in these cases

TABLE 1.   CLINICAL DIAGNOSES IN
EYES WITH NEGATIVE ^{32}P
TEST

Choroidal hemangioma	16
Choroidal nevus	5
Choroidal hematoma	5
Retinal cyst	5
Choroidal pseudotumor	2
Coats's disease	2
Choroidal detachment	2
Subpigment epithelial hemorrhage	1
Pigment epithelial detachment	1
Ectopic disciform detachment	1
Retinal detachment with Von Recklinghausen's disease	1
No diagnosis	5

are listed in Table 1. These patients are being followed, however, and thus far no evidence of an ocular malignancy has appeared in any of them. We definitely feel that a negative ^{32}P test, if correctly performed, is strong evidence against an ocular malignancy.

It is apparent that the most commonly encountered lesion giving a negative ^{32}P test is a choroidal hemangioma, and this constitutes an important disease entity. In many of these cases, prior to the ^{32}P testing, expert clinicians were undecided between the diagnosis of choroidal hemangioma or amelanotic melanoma on the basis of the clinical evaluation. We have found that the ^{32}P test is very useful in making this clinical distinction. Eyes containing choroidal hemangioma are salvageable if the diagnosis is made early, because photocoagulation is effective in clearing the serous detachment and reestablishing central visual acuity.

The next case illustrates the value of a negative ^{32}P test, since it averted an almost certain enucleation. The patient was a 58-year-old white female with a 3-day history of redness and swelling about the left eye with some pain in the eye. She was referred when her local ophthalmologist found a large elevated choroidal mass at the inferonasal border of the optic nerve with a large secondary serous detachment of the retina. The lesion was thought by most observers to be a malignant melanoma of the choroid. A ^{32}P test, however, was negative, and because of this the eye was not enucleated. The patient was treated with subtenons steroid injection. Over the course of the next few weeks, the tumefaction subsided and the serous retinal detachment disappeared. In follow-up over the next 18 months, the patient has been found to have a widespread disturbance of the retinal pigment epithelium, but the choroidal tumor mass is gone and no serous detachment of the retina has reappeared.

SUMMARY

In summary, we have utilized the ^{32}P test in evaluating a total of 231 cases of mass lesions involving the choroid. We feel that this test offers the best means available for differentiating benign from malignant tumors of the choroid. In our experience, false-positive and false-negative test results are rare. Therefore, a positive test is strong evidence that the eye contains a malignancy, while a negative ^{32}P test is strong evidence against the presence of an ocular neoplasm.

REFERENCES

1. Ferry, A. P.: Lesions Mistaken for Malignant Melanoma of the Posterior Uvea. *Arch. Ophthalmol.* **72**:463–469 (1964).

2. Shields, J. A., and Zimmerman, L. E.: Lesions Simulating Malignant Melanoma of the Posterior Uvea. *A.M.A. Arch. Ophthalmol.* **89**:466–471 (1973).

3. Howard, G. M.: Erroneous Clinical Diagnoses of Retinoblastoma and Uveal Melanoma. *Trans. Am. Acad. Ophthalmol. Otolaryng.* **73**:199–203 (1969).

4. Blodi, F. C., and Roy, P. E.: The Misdiagnosed Choroidal Melanoma. *Can. J. Ophthalmol.* **2**:209–211 (1967).

5. Font, R. L., Spaulking, A. G., and Zimmerman, L. E.: Diffuse Malignant Melanoma of the Uveal Tract: A Clinico-Pathologic Report of 54 Cases. *Trans. Am. Acad. Ophthalmol. Otolaryng.* **72**:877–893 (1968).

6. Reese, A. B., and Howard, G. M.: Flat Uveal Melanomas. *Am. J. Ophthalmol.* **64**:1021–1028 (1967).

7. Boniuk, M., and Zimmerman, L. E.: Problems in Differentiating Idiopathic Serous Detachments from Solid Retinal Detachments. *Int. Ophthalmol. Clin.* **2**:411–430 (June 1962).

8. Jarrett, W. H., Green, W. R., Berlin, A. J., and Brawner, J. N.: Retinal Detachment as the Initial Manifestation of Carcinoma of the Lung. *Trans. Am. Acad. Ophthalmol. Otolaryng.* **74**:52–58 (January-February, 1970).

9. Thomas, C. I., Krohmer, J. S. and Storaasli, J. P.: Detection of Intraocular Tumors with Radioactive Phosphorus. *Arch. Ophthalmol.* **47**:276–286 (1952).

10. Dunphy, E. B.: The Role of Radioactive Phosphorus in the Diagnosis of Ocular Malignancy. *Trans. Ophthalmol. Soc. U.K.* **76**:137–152 (1956).

11. Carmichael, P. L., and Leopold, I. H.: The Radioactive Phosphorus Test in Ophthalmology. *Am. J. Ophthalmol.* **49**:484–488 (1960).

12. Leopold, I. H., and Keates, E. U.: Role of Isotopes in Diagnosis of Intraocular Neoplasms. *Trans. Am. Ophthalmol. Soc.* **62**:86–99 (1964).

13. Hagler, W. S., Jarrett, W. H., and Humphrey, W. T.: Radioactive Phosphorus Uptake Test in Diagnosis of Uveal Melanoma. *A.M.A. Arch. Ophthalmol.* **83**:548–557 (1970).

14. Hagler, W. S., Jarrett, W. H., Schnauss, R. H., Larose, J. H., Palms, J. M., and Wood, R. E.: The Diagnosis of Malignant Melanoma of the Ciliary Body or Choroid. *South. Med. J.* **65**:49–54 (January 1972).

^{32}P Testing for Posterior Segment Lesions

Richard S. Ruiz, M.D.
Clinical Professor of Ophthalmology,
University of Texas Medical School,
Houston, Texas

Ernest E. Howerton, Jr., M.D.
Resident in Ophthalmology,
Department of Ophthalmology,
University of Texas Medical School,
Houston, Texas

From the Program in Ophthalmology, The University of Texas Medical School at Houston. Supported by private grant from the Houston Eye Fund.

^{32}P testing introduced to ophthalmology by Thomas et al in 1952[1] has gained wide acceptance as a test for determining the benign or malignant nature of ocular lesions.[2, 3] With experience gained during the first decade, the test was generally thought to be accurate for larger anterior lesions but unreliable in testing smaller posterior lesions.[4, 5] Over the last 10 years, new instruments utilizing modern technological advances have been developed. Greater understanding of the basic properties of ^{32}P and its behavior in benign and malignant tissue has been obtained. Accurate localization, improvements in instrument design, and newer surgical techniques have been employed. All of these factors have transformed ^{32}P testing into a highly accurate and reliable procedure. If done properly, the test is accurate not only for large anterior lesions but also for smaller posterior lesions.[6, 7] This series verifies the reliability of ^{32}P testing if properly performed and correctly interpreted. It also points out the limitations and pitfalls in the procedure.

MATERIALS AND METHODS

In this series of cases radioactive sodium phosphate was given orally in a dose of 10–15 μCi/kg body weight. Readings were delayed for at least 48 hours following administration of dose. All tests were performed with halogen-quenched Geiger-Müller tubes and more recent cases with a solid-state scaler.[8] If the lesion to be tested was located in the ciliary body or anterior choroid, readings were taken in the office through the intact conjunctiva. If the readings were unequivocally positive, no further testing was carried out. If, on the other hand, the readings were borderline or negative, the test was repeated under general anesthesia through a conjunctival incision over the bare sclera and with accurate localization of the lesion. Multiple readings were taken over the lesion and averaged. This figure was compared to the average of multiple readings taken over a normal area in the same eye. The number of readings taken depended on the deviation from the mean and the number of counts per reading. The greater the variation or the lower the counts, the more readings required. As a general rule of procedure, at least six readings should be taken over each area.[9] In our later testing, we have utilized computer analysis of the readings as they are taken to assure statistically valid data and a sufficiently low margin for error. Our arbitrary criterion for positivity has been 100% greater reading over the lesion than the normal area.

This study includes 85 patients who were tested for possible choroidal or ciliary body malignancy. These patients range in age from 9 to 84 years (Fig. 1). No patients were omitted from the study. Eighty cases were tested by one examiner (R. S. R.) and five cases were added through the courtesy of Charles E. Russo, M.D. The percent of ^{32}P uptake versus the malignant or nonmalignant nature of the lesions may be seen in Fig. 2. In this retrospective study, an effort has been made to explore areas of possible misinterpretation of ^{32}P test results.

ANALYSIS OF SERIES

There were 43 cases with readings greater than 100%. Thirty-six of the 43 cases were enucleated and proved to have malignant melanomas of various cell types. One enucleated globe with a reading greater than 100% was diagnosed histologically as containing a metastatic lesion but no primary has been found.

There were seven cases with ^{32}P readings greater than 100% that were not enucleated for various reasons. In one case, the lesion was metastatic from the breast and responded

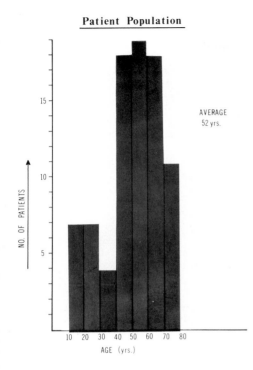

Fig. 1. Population by age.

to radiation. In five cases, although the clinical diagnosis was malignant melanoma, they have only been observed. In one case, the lesion has been treated by photocoagulation because it occurs in a monocular individual.

Of the tests that read below 100%, 14 cases had an averaged reading between 60 and 100% (Fig. 3) and 28 had an averaged reading between zero and 60%. In the 28 cases that read between zero and 60%, the clinical diagnoses included hemangioma of the choroid, disciform lesion, inflammatory lesions of choroid and retina, hyperplasia of the retinal pigment epithelium, and nevus of the choroid. Twenty of the 28 cases read below 30% and only 8 cases read higher. Twelve of those cases with average readings between 60 and 100% are believed to be low-grade malignant melanomas. One case is thought to be a metastatic lesion from the breast, and one case was diagnosed as a retinal angioma.

Forty-three eyes were enucleated (Table 1). Forty enucleated globes had histologically proved malignant melanomas. One eye was histologically diagnosed as containing a metastatic lesion to the choroid but no primary has been found in 4 years of follow-up. In two enucleated eyes the ^{32}P test was negative. The histologic diagnosis was hemangioma of the choroid in one (Figs. 4 and 5) and hemorrhagic disciform lesion in the other (Figs. 6 and 7). Of the 40 enucleated globes that contained malignant melanomas, 36 had ^{32}P readings averaging greater than 100%, while the remaining 4 had readings averaging between 88 and 99%.

DISCUSSION

Throughout this series, the criterion for absolute positivity was 100% or twice as many radioactivity counts over the lesion in a given interval of time compared to readings over

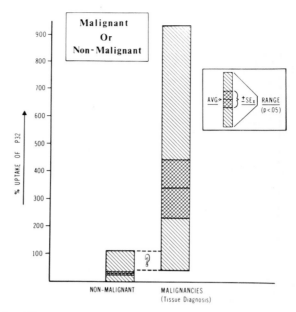

Fig. 2.   Percent uptake of ^{32}P versus clinical and histological diagnoses.

a normal area in the same eye during an equal interval. Using this criterion, there were no false-positive tests. However, as our experience developed, it became apparent that in some cases, with small, flat malignant melanomas of the choroid, this arbitrary criterion was too high. In four cases in which the ^{32}P test was interpreted as positive, the activity ranged between 88 and 99%. The globes were enucleated and found to contain malignant melanomas. In seven additional cases the ^{32}P test ranged from 60 to 88% in eyes that we believe contain small, flat, low-grade malignant melanomas. What is actually needed is a sliding scale of positivity depending on lesion size. It is our general feeling

TABLE 1.   DIAGNOSIS IN 43
ENUCLEATED EYES

Malignant melanoma			40
Mixed cell	21	52.5%	
Spindle A	0	—	
Spindle B	10	25%	
Epithelioid	7	17.5%	
Necrotic	2	5%	
Metastatic disease			1
Adenocarcinoma			
Disciform chorioretinal degeneration			1[a]
Choroidal hemangioma			1[a]
Secondary disciform degeneration			

[a] ^{32}P negative.

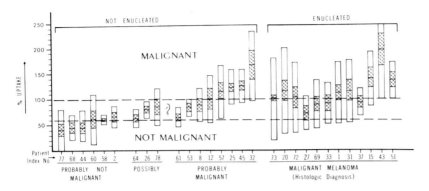

Fig. 3.   Equivocal ^{32}P tests where the range ($p <$ .05) overlaps 60–100% uptake.

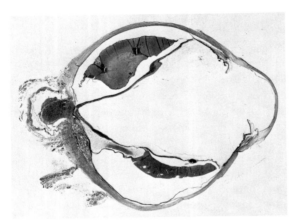

Fig. 4.   Hemangioma of the choroid—low power.

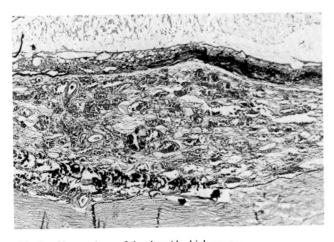

Fig. 5.   Hemangioma of the choroid—high power.

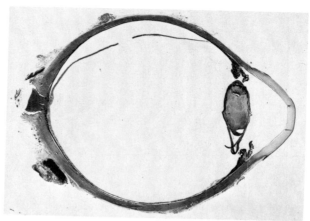

Fig. 6.   Disciform degeneration—low power.

that any lesion 2 mm thick and measuring 6 mm × 6 mm in diameter will read greater than 100% if it is malignant. Based on this experience, no globe should be enucleated with an average reading below 85 percent. It is better to simply observe a small malignant lesion rather than remove an eye unnecessarily. However, if we are to expand the role of ^{32}P testing to diagnose with confidence the benign or malignant nature of small flat lesions, more experience must be gained in testing this type of lesion. It is important that the test be accurately carried out so that meaningful data can be accumulated. With this new information, the malignant nature of small lesions can be verified and early aggressive therapeutic means may then be employed to eradicate the lesion. Radiation plaques and photocoagulation should be more effective on small flat, low-grade malignancies than on large lesions.

In this series no correlation was found between level of ^{32}P reading and cell type of malignant melanoma in enucleated globes (Fig. 8). This does not necessarily mean that no correlation actually exists between level of reading and cell type. However, several

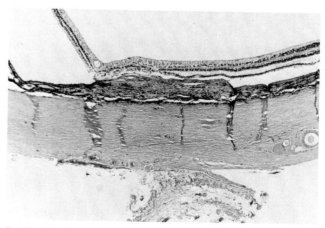

Fig. 7.   Disciform degeneration—high power.

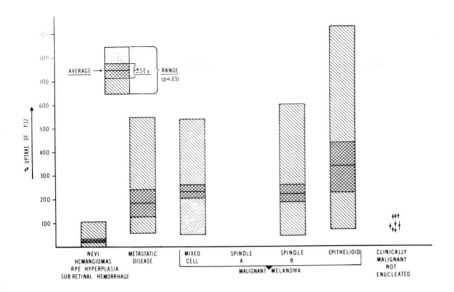

practical points must be considered before trying to analyze this relationship from a retrospective study. The ³²P test as done in the past was considered positive or negative. No attempt was made to obtain maximum readings and accurate statistical data in each case. If the test was unequivocally positive or negative after several readings, further testing was discontinued. Only in those cases in which the test results were borderline was a real effort made to obtain the maximum average readings over the lesion. One can see why a retrospective analysis of cases in an attempt to correlate cell type and number of counts would be uncertain. A prospective study with painstaking technique to obtain maximum counts in each case would be necessary for an accurate analysis. In addition, computer analysis of the counts during the testing would be required to assure reasonable tolerance levels and statistically valid data. We feel that our present techniques and instruments are sufficiently crude to make this a very doubtful undertaking.

Based on our experience, we feel there is good reason to doubt Callender's classification of cell type as a reliable index of the degree of malignancy. It is quite possible that an accurately performed ³²P test may give a more sensitive index of the degree of malignancy based on the level of reading.

Two eyes were enucleated in spite of negative ³²P studies. In one eye, there was a total retinal detachment with an underlying elevated pigmented mass and no light perception. This was proven to be a choroidal hemangioma (Figs. 4 and 5). In this case the ³²P reading was definitely negative, averaging 6% greater over the lesion than a normal area in the same eye. The second negative ³²P study in which the eye was enucleated proved to be a massive eccentric hemorrhagic disciform lesion (Figs. 6 and 7). The patient was seen originally with a large, dark, highly elevated subretinal mass which involved almost one quadrant of the fundus. ³²P testing was negative with a reading 10% greater over the lesion than the normal area. Clinical diagnosis at that time was a massive spontaneous subretinal hemorrhage from the choroid. Blood subsequently ruptured through the retina into the vitreous, making further visualization of the fundus impossible. The patient was followed for a period of 10 months and lost all useful vision. It was the consensus of opinion that the safest course was to remove the globe. The histologic diagnosis was hemorrhagic disciform lesion of the choroid.

In this series, there were four hemangiomas of the choroid. One occurred in a 9-year-old boy in which the original diagnosis was malignant melanoma of the choroid. The ^{32}P test, however, read only 8% higher over the lesion. On the basis of this negative study, the lesion was treated with diathermy and photocoagulation. The secondary detachment disappeared, and he has been followed now for 5 years with no sign of recurrence or growth. Another choroidal hemangioma has been cited earlier in this report with histologic confirmation. In another case, the clinical diagnosis was hemangioma of the choroid and readings were 20% higher over the lesion. In only one instance did a vascular lesion read greater than 50%. In this case, there was a highly elevated ball-like lesion which measured 6 mm × 6 mm. It protruded from the retinal surface into the vitreous. At the time of our original examination, the lesion had already been treated with intensive photocoagulation, and there was chorioretinal scarring around the base of the lesion. With fluorescein angiography the lesion lit up intensely in the retinal arterial phase, demonstrating that it was largely composed of blood vessels from the retinal circulation. ^{32}P readings over the lesion averaged 61% higher than the normal area. Within the substance of the lesion were accumulations of white exudative-like material which was believed to be white blood cells. Perhaps this contributed to the increased readings since white blood cells have been shown to assimilate ^{32}P. However, a malignant lesion 6 mm × 6 mm × 6 mm in dimension would be expected to read well over 100%.

Several inflammatory lesions were tested. One typical toxoplasmic lesion read 0% greater uptake. Another case diagnosed as peripheral uveitis with heavy exudative material over the pars plana and peripheral retina below read 10%.

One final case deserves special mention because the ^{32}P test was interpreted as negative and subsequently the eye proved to have a metastatic lesion. This eye had been operated upon on two previous occasions for retinal detachment. At the time of our evaluation, the entire lower choroid, anterior to the equator, was destroyed by previous diathermy and cryotherapy. The lower half of the retina was detached and gliotic. There was no elevated lesion visible beneath the detached retina, and the choroid in the posterior pole region appeared normal. It was my firm clinical impression that there was no neoplastic lesion present, but a ^{32}P study was recommended and an attempt to repair the retinal detachment if the test was negative. One of the prime requisites of the testing procedure was violated because there was no definite lesion to test and compare against normal. In addition, the globe had been subjected to previous surgery on two occasions and the sclera and external surface were markedly thickened and scarred in some areas while being very thin to the point of exposed bare choroid in others. The readings were taken in a survey manner comparing the lower abnormal to the upper normal half of the globe. Readings averaged 80% higher below than above. The test was interpreted as negative but the patient subsequently proved to have a metastatic choroidal lesion from the breast.

It is imperative to understand that many facets of ^{32}P testing are purely empirical in nature, for example, dose, delay in reading, and criteria for positivity. Many of the sources for unreliability in early testing stem from erroneous concepts or lack of understanding of the basic nature and limitations of the test. It is easy to understand why the test was lauded for large lesions. Basic knowledge of the radiation characteristics of ^{32}P indicate that the beta particle only travels an average of 3 mm in tissue.[10] Therefore, in a large anterior lesion which perhaps fills a quadrant, the probe can easily be placed over the lesion almost blindly without any conjunctival incision or localization. If the conjunctiva is incised and the probe placed on the bare sclera, accuracy may be enhanced. However, posterior smaller lesions must be very accurately localized to ensure proper probe placement directly over the lesion. This extremely important concept was emphasized by Hagler et al[7] in 1969.

With proper localization and direct exposure of the sclera over the lesion, it is desirable to use a different probe design for maximum accuracy. Because of the short tissue traveling distance of the beta particle, one can appreciate that sliding on the surface of the sclera or tilting the probe face during the counting interval may result in inaccurate counts and erroneous interpretation. Obviously, the smaller the lesion the more important are these factors. For this reason a serrated border has been placed around the face for gripping purposes.[8]

Dosage of ^{32}P has been purely arbitrary at 10 μCi/kg body weight.[7] The medication has routinely been given intravenously; however, our experience has shown that oral administration of this same dosage level is quite reliable and much easier. Sodium phosphate is an odorless, colorless, tasteless liquid in no way offensive to the patient. In addition, with the oral route there is no problem of contamination or extravasation.

The time of reading following administration of the dose has varied since the test was initially introduced. Originally readings were taken at 1 hour and 24 hours,[1, 11, 12] then a 48-hour reading was added. The 48-hour reading was subsequently found to be more accurate than either the 1- or 24-hour reading.[12] However, the ideal time to count radioactivity in a malignant melanoma after administration of the dose is still not known. We have had occasion to read at 48 hours and repeat at 13 days. The counts were equally high at the latter time. This delay in reading becomes extremely important with vascular lesions; also, low-grade, small, malignant lesions probably require longer to maximally assimilate ^{32}P within the nuclear protein because of slower mitotic activity. There should be an optimum time to count which considers the half-life of ^{32}P, the time necessary for maximum absorption of the isotope by the lesion, and the time of maximum clearing of the vascular system and normal tissue.

Another error in early testing was to use the fellow eye as control.[13, 14] Needless to say, with the short tissue traveling distance of the beta particle, the ideal control is a known normal area in the same eye. Reports of the unreliability of ^{32}P testing in postoperative eyes stems from the fact that the fellow eye was used as control. This simply points out that increased vascularity will increase the reading, as will white blood cells, both of which would be nullified if a specific lesion were being tested against a known normal area in the same eye.

If the test is viewed simply as a comparison of normal to abnormal, one can readily appreciate the danger in testing eyes with opaque media or where a specific normal and abnormal area cannot be identified.

CONCLUSION

We feel that radioactive phosphorous testing is an extremely reliable and accurate means of determining whether an ocular lesion is malignant or benign. It is of utmost importance that the test be properly performed and that the radiation characteristics, the limitations, and the pitfalls involved in the test be adequately understood. There are many basic facets of the test that need to be elucidated, for example the optimum dosage, the ideal testing time, an accurate sliding scale of positivity relative to lesion size, and testing procedure, which will lead to statistically valid conclusions in each individual test. With these improvements and increased accuracy in diagnosing small, flat melanomas, early aggressive local therapy can then be confidently undertaken to destroy the lesion, save the globe, and perhaps, in some cases, restore useful vision.

REFERENCES

1. Thomas, C. I., Krohmer, J. S., and Storaasli, P.: Detection of Intraocular Tumors with Radioactive Phosphorus: A Preliminary Report with Special Reference to Differentiation of the Cause of Retinal Separation. *Arch. Ophthalmol.* **47**:276 (1952).

2. Terner, I. S., Lepold, I. H., and Eisenberg, I. J.: The Radioactive Phosphorus (^{32}P) Uptake Test in Ophthalmology. *Arch. Ophthalmol.* **55**:52–80 (1956).

3. Hagler, W. S., Jarrett, W. H. II, and Humphrey, W. T.: The Radioactive Phosphorus Uptake Test in Diagnosis of Uveal Melanoma. *Arch. Ophthalmol.* (Chicago) **83**:548–57 (May 1970).

4. Donn, A., and McTigue, J. W.: The Radioactive Phosphorus Uptake Test for Malignant Melanoma of the Eye. *Arch. Ophthalmol.* **57**:668–671 (1957).

5. O'Rourke, J., and Collins, E.: ^{32}P Localization of Malignant Melanoma of the Posterior Choroid. *Arch. Ophthalmol.* **63**:81–91 (1960).

6. Ruiz, R. S., McGehee, F. O., and Allen, H. C.: A New Technique of ^{32}P Testing of Lesions of the Posterior Segment. *South. Med. J.* **65** (7):(1972).

7. Hagler, W. S., Jarrett, W. H. II, Schnauss, R. H., LaRose, J. S., Palms, J. M., and Wood, R. E.: The Diagnosis of Malignant Melanoma of the Ciliary Body or Choroid: Use of the Radioactive Phosphorus Uptake Test. *South. Med. J.* **65** (1):(January 1972).

8. Ruiz, R. S.: New Radioactivity Detection Probe and Scaler for Phosphorus-32 Testing of Ocular Lesions. *Trans. Am. Acad. Ophthalmol. Otolaryngol.* **76**:535–536 (1972).

9. Ruiz, R. S., and Howerton, E. E., Jr.: Choroidal Melanoma Size and Accuracy with ^{32}P Testing. *Am. J. Ophthalmol.* (in press).

10. Bettman, J. W.: Radioactive Isotopes. *Arch. Ophthalmol.* **59**:821–831 (1958).

11. Eisenberg, I. J., Terner, I. S., and Leopold, I. H.: Use of ^{32}P as an Aid in Diagnosis of Intraocular Neoplasms. *Arch. Ophthalmol.* **52**:741–750 (1954).

12. Goldberg, B., Tabowitz, D., Kara, G. B., Zarell, S., and Espiritv, R.: The Use of ^{32}P in the Diagnosis of Ocular Tumors. *Arch. Ophthalmol.* **65**:68–83 (1961).

13. Eisenberg, I. J., Leopold, I. H., and Sklaroff, D.: Use of Radioactive Phosphorus in Detection of Intraocular Neoplasms. *Arch. Ophthalmol.* **51**:633–641 (1954).

14. Dunphy, E. B., Dowling, J. L., and Scott, A.: Experience with Radioactive Phosphorus in Tumor Detection. *Trans. Am. Ophthalmol. Soc.* **54** (1956).

The Radioactive Phosphorus Uptake Test in the Diagnosis of Ocular Tumors

Jerry A. Shields, M.D.
Senior Assistant Surgeon,
Retina Service,
Wills Eye Hospital,
Philadelphia, Pennsylvania

Paul L. Carmichael, M.D.
Clinical Associate Professor,
Department of Radiation Therapy
and Nuclear Medicine,
Hahnemann Medical College;
Assistant Surgeon, Retina Service,
Wills Eye Hospital,
Philadelphia, Pennsylvania

Brian C. Leonard, M.D., FRCS (C)
Assistant Professor of Ophthalmology,
University of Ottawa,
Ottawa, Canada

Jay L. Federman, M.D.
Senior Assistant Surgeon,
Wills Eye Hospital;
Assistant Professor of Ophthalmology,
Thomas Jefferson University,
Philadelphia, Pennsylvania

Lov K. Sarin, M.D.
Attending Surgeon,
Retina Service,
Wills Eye Hospital;
Clinical Professor of Ophthalmology,
Thomas Jefferson University,
Philadelphia, Pennsylvania

The difficulties in the clinical diagnosis of uveal melanomas are well known to ophthalmologists.[1, 2] A recent report indicates that these difficulties may be greatly alleviated by the utilization of certain diagnostic modalities now available.[3] Perhaps the most widely acclaimed diagnostic adjunct is the radioactive phosphorus uptake test (^{32}P). Although this test was once widely used, it fell into disfavor for several years, until a recent report stimulated renewed interest in the procedure.[4] Its renewed popularity has been largely due to improved instrumentation and the introduction of better probes for counting lesions located in the posterior segment of the globe.[4, 5, 6] Several recent reports have stressed the great reliability of this test when carefully performed.[7-13]

When the lesion is located in the anterior segment of the globe, it is not necessary to perform an incision to perform the test. If the lesion is located in the posterior segment, however, a surgical approach must be utilized.[7] This report discusses the accuracy of the ^{32}P test as determined from a series of 300 consecutive tests. This first section considers the nonsurgical, or transconjunctival, approach, and the second section will discuss the surgical, or transcleral, technique.

MATERIALS AND METHODS

A total of 300 ^{32}P tests performed by the Oncology Unit, Retina Service, Wills Eye Hospital, are the subject of this report. The study comprised a 4-year period extending from February 1971 to February 1975. Most tests were performed by, or under the supervision of, a single investigator (JAS), and all were performed with strict adherence to techniques described in the literature.[4, 7, 15] In most instances, both the Geiger-Müller counter and the solid-state semiconductor detector unit were used to perform the procedure (Fig. 1). All transconjunctival (nonsurgical) tests were first analyzed to determine the diagnostic accuracy of the procedure for tumors located in the anterior segment of the globe. A positive test was interpreted as one showing an uptake of greater than 30% over the control area at 1 hour after injection, with an increasing uptake during the next 48 hours. The control area was usually the symmetric quadrant of the opposite eye.

All tests performed by the transcleral (surgical) route were then analyzed in a similar manner to determine the accuracy of the procedure for tumors located in the posterior segment of the globe. A positive test was considered as an uptake of greater than 50% over the control area at 48 hours after injection. The control area was the opposite quadrant of the same eye.

The cases were analyzed with regard to accuracy of this test in differentiating benign from malignant lesions. Those cases showing false negative or false positive results were selected for closer scrutiny in order to gain insight into reasons for false results.

RESULTS

I. Transconjunctival Route

The 300 consecutive ^{32}P tests in this study were performed by the Oncology Unit of the Retina Service of the Wills Eye Hospital between February 1971 and February 1975.

From the Oncology Unit, Retina Service, Wills Eye Hospital, Philadelphia. Supported in part by the Retina Research and Development Foundation, Philadelphia, and the Lions Club of Pennsylvania.

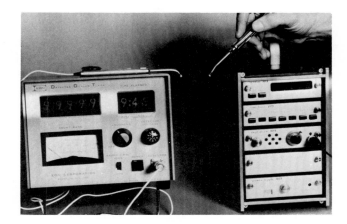

Fig. 1. Instruments utilized in performing the ^{32}P test. Left: The Detector Ocular Tumor unit (EON Corporation). Right: The solid-state semiconductor detector (Nuclear Associates; Technical Associates). The probes utilized are illustrated above the instruments.

The general statistics regarding these tests are shown in Table 1. In four cases, the test was performed twice on one lesion several months apart; in five cases, the test was later repeated after a lesion had been treated locally. The 300 tests, therefore, were performed on a total of 291 patients, but this discrepancy does not significantly change any of the involved statistics. As illustrated in Table 1, 106 procedures were done by the transconjunctival technique and 8 cases were performed by both the transconjunctival and transcleral routes. A total of 114 cases, therefore, were performed by the transconjunctival method.

A further breakdown of these 114 cases is shown in Table 2. There were 64 positive tests and 50 negative tests. Of the 64 positive tests, 60 were histologically confirmed. All 60 of these were malignant melanomas, and there were no histologically confirmed false-positive tests. Of the 4 cases that were not confirmed, 3 were clear-cut cases of metastatic malignant tumors which were treated by irradiation at other institutions. The only positive test that was felt to be nonmalignant was a patient who had a presumed spontaneous choroidal hemorrhage at the time of cataract surgery, which simulated a malignant melanoma. The transconjunctival test was positive 4 days after cataract surgery. The test was negative, however, when repeated by the transcleral route 6 weeks after surgery.

There were 50 negative tests by the transconjunctival technique. Four of these were histologically confirmed as malignant melanomas of the anterior segment and must be classified as false negative tests. Four other cases were diagnosed clinically as probable iris melanomas, but are being followed conservatively for one reason or another. These should be classified as *possible* false-negative tests. One small peripheral choroidal tumor, which gave a negative test, was believed clinically to be a small melanoma and should also be considered a *possible* false-negative, although the lesion has not grown in a 1-year follow-up period. The final false-negative case was a metastatic tumor located in the equatorial region where the probe could not be accurately placed. The diagnoses for the remainder of the negative tests are shown in Table 2. Thorough clinical studies and follow-up evaluation from 1 to 4 years have clearly shown that these lesions are not malignant. With the transconjunctival technique, we found no significant difference between the two standard instruments used.

TABLE 1. GENERAL STATISTICS ON 300 CONSECUTIVE ^{32}P TESTS FOR SUSPECTED OCULAR TUMORS

Total tests		300
Transconjunctival (noncutting) route		106
Positive	57	
Negative	49	
Transcleral (cutting) route		186
Positive	127	
Negative	59	
Both transconjunctival and transcleral route		8
Positive both routes	6	
Negative both routes	1	
Positive transconjunctival, negative transcleral	1	

TABLE 2. DISTRIBUTION AND DIAGNOSES FOR ^{32}P TESTS PERFORMED BY THE TRANSCONJUNCTIVAL ROUTE

Total tests			114
Positive			64
Histologically confirmed		60	
Iris and/or ciliary body			
Malignant melanoma	56		
Metastatic tumor	3		
Conjunctival malignant melanoma	1		
Not histologically confirmed		4	
Metastatic tumors	3		
Choroidal hemorrhage	1		
(Same case later negative with transcleral approach)			
Negative			50
Histologically confirmed		4	
Iris malignant melanoma	3		
Ciliary body malignant melanoma	1		
Not Histologically confirmed		46	
Iris nevus	19		
Iris malignant melanoma	4		
Iris or ciliary body cyst	4		
Vitreous hemorrhage	5		
Choroidal effusion	2		
Choroidal hemorrhage	2		
Heterochromia	2		
Ectopic disciform degeneration	2		
Choroidal melanoma	1		
Hypertrophy, RPE	1		
Serous Retinal Detachment	1		
Metastatic tumor	1		
Absolute glaucoma	1		
Granuloma	1		

For the 114 cases of transconjunctival ^{32}P tests, therefore, there was only one possible false-positive test, for an incidence of less than 1%. Of the 114 cases, the number of false-negative tests is between 4 and 10 for an incidence between 3.5% and 9%. The reasons for false results will be considered shortly.

II. Transcleral Route

Of the 300 ^{32}P tests performed by the Oncology Unit of the Retina Service of Wills Eye Hospital in this series, 186 were performed by the transcleral route alone and 8 were performed by both the transconjunctival and transcleral routes, making a total of 194 tests performed by the transcleral technique (Table 2). There were 132 positive tests and 62 negative tests (Table 3).

Of the 132 tests that were positive, 107 were histologically confirmed. This included 105 cases of malignant melanoma and 2 cases of metastatic tumor. The diagnoses are listed for the 25 positive tests that were not histologically confirmed. Twenty of these

TABLE 3. DISTRIBUTION AND DIAGNOSIS FOR ^{32}P TESTS PERFORMED BY THE TRANSCLERAL ROUTE

Total tests					194
Positive				132	
Histologically confirmed			107		
Malignant melanoma		105			
Metastatic tumor		2			
Not histologically confirmed			25		
Malignant melanoma		20			
Photocoagulated	8				
Being followed	6				
Refused surgery	3				
Lost to follow-up	2				
Irradiated	1				
Metastatic tumor		5			
Negative				62	
Histologically confirmed			5		
Malignant melanoma	4				
Choroidal hemangioma	1				
Not histologically confirmed			57		
Choroidal nevus (possible small malignant melanoma)	18				
Choroidal hemangioma	13				
Malignant melanoma previously treated by photocoagulation	5				
Serous retinal detachment	4				
Disciform maculopathy	4				
Retinal/choroidal hemorrhage	4				
Chorioretinitis	3				
Vitreous hemorrhage	3				
Astrocytoma	2				
Retinal vein occlusion	1				

were small melanomas which were diagnosed by clinical appearance, visual fields, fluorescein angiography, and ultrasonography, leaving no doubt in our opinion, as to their true diagnosis. Eight were treated with photocoagulation, one with cobalt irradiation, and the others were not treated for one reason or another. Five cases were well-documented metastatic tumors which were treated with irradiation and/or chemotherapy at another institution. There were no documented false-positive tests.

There were 62 negative tests by the transcleral route. Five of the 62 were histologically confirmed. Four were malignant melanomas and therefore, represented false negative tests. One case was a choroidal hemangioma which was subsequently enucleated despite a negative ^{32}P test. This case has been reported elsewhere.[8]

There were 57 negative cases that were not histologically confirmed. The diagnoses are listed. Eighteen of these were suspicious choroidal nevi which have so far shown no growth during a 1- to 4-year follow-up period. Thirteen were well-documented cases of choroidal hemangiomas which were referred for the ^{32}P test to rule out an amelanotic melanoma.

Five tests were performed upon choroidal melanoma cases where the tumor had been treated several times with xenon photocoagulation. In every instance, the test converted from positive to negative following presumed eradication of the tumor. These cases are the subject of a separate report.[17] The remaining negative tests included a variety of lesions clinically diagnosed as benign and documented upon follow-up studies. For the most part, the readings of the two instruments were consistent, and we found no significant advantage of one unit over the other.

Of the 194 cases on which the transcleral ^{32}P test was performed, there were no documented false-positive tests and only 4 documented false-negative tests. The incidence of false negative tests, therefore, is about 2%.

DISCUSSION

Following the introduction of the ^{32}P test into ophthalmology,[14] most of the early workers utilized primarily the transconjunctival approach for all suspicious lesions regardless of their location in the globe.[15, 16] False-negative results were frequent because the probe could not be placed near enough to the base of the lesion to be evaluated. Our experience has shown that the transconjunctival approach can be reliable only in those cases where the lesion is *anterior* in the globe, involving the iris and/or ciliary body (Fig. 2). In some small, flat, iris lesions, however, false-negative results may occur (Fig. 3). In addition, some small peripheral choroidal lesions, even though the lesion can be reached with routine scleral depression, may give a false-negative result. One must incise the conjunctiva in the latter instances.

Radioactive phosphorus emits beta particles, which travel only an average of 4 mm through tissue, so it is feasible that intervening cornea, aqueous, ciliary body, or angle structures might decrease the particles reaching the window of the probe. This probably explained the negative test obtained in four histologically confirmed iris melanomas in this series.

This study tends to support the important role of the transcleral ^{32}P test for *posterior* uveal melanomas. In 194 tests performed by this technique, there were no false-positive results and only four false-negatives. In our experience, most choroidal melanomas greater than 1.5 mm in elevation and 3 mm in diameter, will give a positive test when the procedure is carefully performed[7] (Figs. 4 and 5). The false-negative tests can be

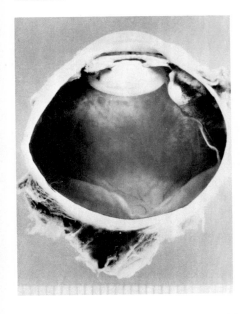

Fig. 2. Malignant melanoma arising from ciliary body and extending to iris and choroid. This lesion gave a strongly positive ^{32}P test by the transconjunctival approach.

explained on the basis of the size and location of the tumor. Two of the false-negative tests were due to small lesions which grew around the termination of Bruch's membrane to protrude anteriorly over the optic nerve head. Since the optic nerve is about 3 mm in diameter posterior to the globe, and only 1.5 mm in diameter at the optic disc, it becomes technically difficult in such cases to place the window of the probe over the base of the tumor (Fig. 6).

In two cases, the false-negative tests were due to small spindle-cell melanomas in the posterior choroid. These, however, were borderline false-negative tests. In a large series such as this, it is not surprising that an occasional borderline case will be encountered. We must acknowledge that some of the suspicious pigmented lesions that gave a nega-

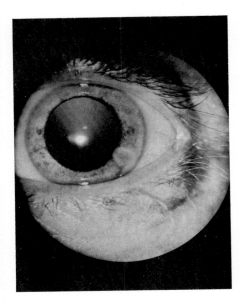

Fig. 3. Small, relatively flat iris melanoma that gave a false negative ^{32}P test.

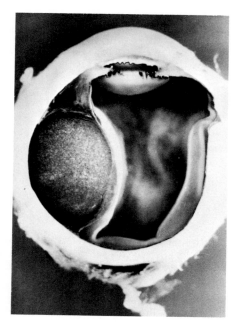

Fig. 4.   Large equatorial melanoma. This lesion gave a strongly positive result (500%) when transcleral ^{32}P test was performed.

tive test may be early malignant melanomas of the choroid. This may not be a matter of great clinical significance, however, since small choroidal melanomas are usually slow growing and offer a relatively good prognosis.[2] In such cases, a period of observation for signs of growth may be the proper approach.

Most of the lesions producing negative results were clear-cut cases of benign lesions which are known to occasionally simulate melanomas.[1, 2] Follow-up studies from 1 to 4 years have thus far substantiated the benign nature of these lesions.

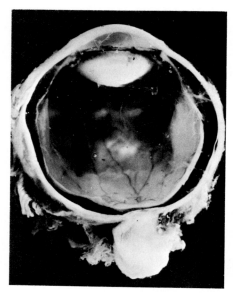

Fig. 5.   Small melanoma in posterior pole that gave a positive result (200%) when transcleral ^{32}P test was performed.

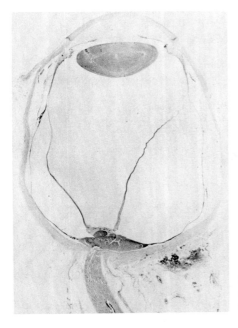

Fig. 6. Small choroidal melanoma protruding anteriorly over optic nerve head gave a false negative ^{32}P test due to difficulty in placing probe over base of lesion.

SUMMARY

Of the 300 consecutive ^{32}P tests performed by the Oncology Unit, Retina Service, Wills Eye Hospital, 106 were done by the transconjunctival route, 186 by the transcleral route, and 8 by both routes. With the transconjunctival (noncutting) technique, the incidence of documented false-positive results was less than 1% and the incidence of documented false negative results was 3.5%. With the transcleral (cutting) technique, there were no false-positive results and an incidence of 2% false-negative results. It is concluded that the ^{32}P test, when properly performed, is probably the most accurate ancillary test now available for differentiating benign from malignant intraocular lesions.

REFERENCES

1. Ferry, A. P.: Lesions Mistaken for Malignant Melanomas of the Posterior Uvea. *Arch. Ophthalmol.* **72**:463 (1964).
2. Shields, J. A., and Zimmerman, L. E.: Lesions Simulating Malignant Melanomas of the Posterior Uvea. *Arch. Ophthalmol.* **89**:466 (1973).
3. Shields, J. A., and McDonald, P. R.: Improvements in the Diagnosis of Posterior Uveal Melanomas. *Trans. Am. Ophthalmol. Soc.* **71**:193 (1973); *Arch. Ophthalmol.* **91**:259 (1974).
4. Hagler, W. S., Jarrett, W. H. II, and Humphrey, W. T.: The Radioactive Phosphorus Uptake Test in the Diagnosis of Uveal Melanomas. *Arch. Ophthalmol.* **83**:548 (1970).
5. Hagler, W. S., Jarrett, W. H. II, Schnauss, R. H. et al: The Diagnosis of Malignant Melanoma of the Ciliary Body or Choroid. Use of the Radioactive Phosphorus Uptake Test. *South. Med. J.* **65**:49 (1972).
6. Ruiz, R. S.: New Radioactivity Detection Probe and Scaler for Phosphorus-32 Testing of Ocular Lesions. *Trans. Am. Acad. Ophthalmol. Otolaryngol.* **76**:535 (1972).
7. Shields, J. A., Sarin, L. K., Federman, J. L., Mensheha-Manhart, O., and Carmichael, P. L.: Surgical Approach to the ^{32}P Test for Posterior Uveal Melanomas. *Ophthalmol. Surg.* **5**:13 (1974).

8. Shields, J. A., Hagler, W. S., Federman, J. L., Jarrett, W. H. II, and Carmichael, P. L.: The Significance of the ^{32}P Uptake Test in the Diagnosis of Posterior Uveal Melanomas. *Trans. Am. Acad. Ophthalmol. Otolaryngol.* (in press).

9. Carmichael, P. L., Holst, G. C., Federman, J. L., and Shields, J. A.: The Present Status of the ^{32}P Test in Ophthalmology. In Croll, M., Ed., *New Techniques in Tumor Localization and Radioimmunoassay.* John Wiley, New York, 1974.

10. Shields, J. A., Carmichael, P. L., Leonard, B. C., Federman, J. L., and Sarin, L. K.: The Accuracy of the ^{32}P Test for Ocular Melanomas. Presented at the AMA Section on Ophthalmology, June 16, 1975 (submitted for publication).

11. Shields, J. A., Annesley, W. H. Jr., and Totino, J. A.: Nonfluorescent Malignant Melanoma of the Choroid Diagnosed with the ^{32}P Test. *Am. J. Ophthalmol.* **79**:634 (1975).

12. Shields, J. A., Leonard, B. C., and Sarin, L. K.: Multinodular Uveal Melanoma Masquerading as a Postoperative Choroidal Detachment (in preparation).

13. Shields, J. A., and McDonald, P. R.: Ultrasound and ^{32}P in the Diagnosis of Melanomas with Opaque Media (in preparation).

14. Thomas, C. I., Krohmer, J. S., and Storaasli, J. P.: Detection of Intraocular Tumors with Radioactive Phosphorus: A Preliminary Report with Special Reference to Differentiation of the Cause of Retinal Separation. *Arch. Ophthalmol.* **47**:276 (1952).

15. Carmichael, P. L., and Leopold, I. H.: Radioactive Phosphorus Test in Ophthalmology. *Am. J. Ophthalmol.* **49**:484 (1960).

16. Leopold, I. H., Keates, E. U., and Charkes, I. D.: Role of Isotopes in Diagnosis of Intraocular Neoplasm. *Trans. Am. Ophthalmol. Soc.* **42**:86 (1964).

17. Shields, J. A., Annesley, W. H. Jr., Sarin, L. K., and Federman, J. L.: Fluorescein and ^{32}P Studies in Photocoagulated Choroidal Melanomas. Presented at Atlantic Section, Association for Research in Vision and Ophthalmology, Bethesda, November 2, 1974 (in preparation for publication).

Limitations of the ^{32}P Test for Detection of Choroidal Melanoma

Ijaz Shafi, M.D.
Assistant Professor of Ophthalmology,
University of Connecticut Health Center,
Division of Ophthalmology,
Farmington, Connecticut

James F. O'Rourke, M.D.
Professor and Chairman,
Department of Ophthalmology,
Cornell University School of Medicine,
Manhattan, New York

Donald P. D'Amato, Ph.D.
Assistant Professor of Ophthalmology,
Division of Ophthalmology,
University of Connecticut Health Center,
Farmington, Connecticut

Gehangir Durrani, M.D.
Assistant Professor of Ophthalmology,
Division of Ophthalmology,
University of Connecticut Health
Center;
Chief of Ophthalmology,
Veterans Hospital,
Farmington, Connecticut

Recommendations for the ^{32}P test have for many years stressed its limitations, based principally upon difficulties of in vivo beta counting.[1, 2, 3] This report presents our divergent views concerning eye tumor management and the place of ^{32}P counting.

The counting procedure must employ the highest count rate that is practical over the tumor bed and a reference area. The test has a firm mathematical basis, as does any counting procedure. Unfortunately, the count rate may be abnormally low and short counting periods are common. Long counting times in the operating room with a handheld detector are needed but may introduce geometric errors. A clamp, similar to the one shown in Fig. 1, when attached to the operating table aids in positioning the probe against the exposed sclera. The operating room staff must be made aware of the longer time requirement so that the high totals needed can be obtained.

Once the eye has been enucleated, a "moment of truth" count should be obtained over the transilluminated tumor bed (Fig. 2). Tracer incorporated into the tumor cells does not leave after enucleation. The near perfect counting geometry now available offers the best possible evaluation of the test. This counting rate and total, plus those of the measurement before enucleation and the tumor size ought to be recorded and given in published reports. It is the long-term evaluation of these numbers, rather than of percent increases, that will determine the value of the test and others to follow.

A frozen section of the tumor taken in the pathology laboratory immediately after surgery, with the surgeon present, is in our opinion desirable. This need not interfere with subsequent processing of the specimen. It provides the patient and family with a prompt diagnosis and prognosis.

A nonnuclear method for differentiating melanoma from hemangioma, subretinal hemorrhage, or serous detachment, which in our hands has proven most useful, has been the infrared fundus photograph. It has the effect of transillumination of the posterior fundus regions, without the need for surgical exposure. It is a sensitive method for following the progress of suspected melanomas, since the borders are sharply defined. These features appear in color in Figs. 3a and b. The initial use of this film for fundus photography was reported by Ernest in 1968. However, since that time its adoption by retinal surgeons for the study of solid detachments has apparently been rather limited.

Infrared film* is used in the fundus camera along with a Kodak Wratten #12 filter (medium yellow). This is a modified color reversal type film consisting of three image layers, sensitive to infrared, red, and green. (The layers are also sensitive to blue light which is subtracted by the filter.) The film is processed by the readily available Kodak E-4 process. Retina and blood are mostly transparent to the longer red and infrared wavelengths recorded by the film. For this reason, hemangioma and subretinal hemorrhage are obliterated. Melanin pigment, on the other hand, displays a marked absorption of these rays. To visualize a pigmented mass beneath the retina, use of an infrared sensitive emulsion is indicated. We have been most impressed with the value of Dr. Ernest's method when used to identify and document the growth of choroidal melanoma.

A final note on the management of melanoma concerns the clinical interpretations to be placed on current pathological reports dealing with cell type, prognosis, avoiding unnecessary enucleation, and so forth. There is reason to believe that many more patients die with metastases after enucleation than we had heretofore suspected. Our preoccupa-

* Eastman Kodak Co, IE 135-20.

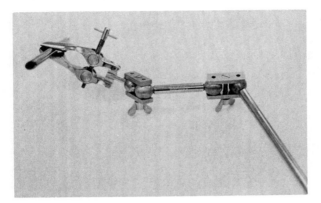

Fig. 1.   Clamp to hold and position ^{32}P probe in operating room.

tion with the need to avoid enucleation mistakes ought to emphasize a need for more accurate and earlier diagnosis. It should not cause a casual approach to cancer management. The basis of these remarks is Jensen's impressive, though little noted, report in 1970 of long-term follow-up of enucleated patients in Denmark.[4] Jensen found that 154 of 292 patients (53%) died with metastasis within 15 years of enucleation. Among 83 spindle-cell types (74B;9A), 24 died with metastases; among 111 mixed cell types, 96 died with metastases; and of 26 epitheloid type, 21 died with metastases. His figures are based on autopsy, laparotomy, biopsy, and death certificate reports. They do not encourage the view that enucleation, as now scheduled, is highly curative for any cell type. Jensen's evidence, and other's, indicates that enucleation of tumors sized below 10 mm × 10 mm, or five disc diameters, gives improved prognosis. This may mean that earlier rather than later enucleation is indicated.

In our opinion, irrespective of the size of the mass, once growth is documented by serial fundus infrared photography, the surgeon should recommend a ^{32}P study with

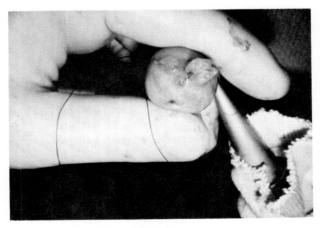

Fig. 2.   Transillumination of enucleated eye.

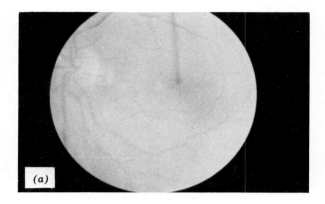

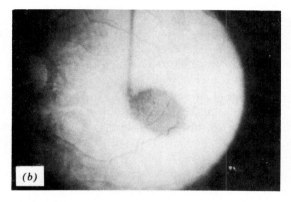

Fig. 3. (a) Conventional fundus photograph of pigmented lesion. (b) Infrared modified photograph of the same region as shown in (a).

enucleation if positive, and enucleation soon thereafter if the ^{32}P test is negative and growth continues. We do not believe that slow growth observed in many tumors is evidence against metastases. The two processes (growth and metastases) are not necessarily related. Therefore, if the mass is pigmented and it grows (as shown by infrared studies), remove it, and the smaller the better.

REFERENCES

1. O'Rourke, J., Patton, H., and Bradley, B.: Fundamental Limitations of Radiophosphorus Counting Methods Used for Detection of Intraocular Melanomas. *Arch. Ophthalmol.* **57**:730–738 (1957).

2. O'Rourke, J., and Collins, E.: P-32 Localization of Malignant Melanoma of the Posterior Choroid. *Arch. Ophthalmol.* **63**:801–811 (1960).

3. O'Rourke, J., and D'Amato, D. P.: Counting Statistics Required for [32]P Detection of Choroidal Melanoma. *Arch. Ophthalmol.* (in press); correspondence (1975).

4. Jensen, O. A.: Malignant Melanomas of the Human Uvea; Recent Follow-Up of Cases in Denmark (1943–52) *Acta Ophthalmol.* **48**:1113–1128 (1970).

Lesions of
the Uvea

NONCONTACT DETECTION

Application of the Cerenkov Effect for the Detection of Endocular Tumors

N. Safi, M.D.
Hôpital Pellegrin,
Service des Isotopes,
Place Amelie Raba-Leon,
Bordeaux, France

P. Blanquet, M.D.
Director, de L'Unite de Recherches,
Inserm,
Bordeaux, France

M. J. LeRebeller, M.D.
Service d'Ophthalmologie,
Hôpital Saint-Andre,
Bordeaux, France

D. Blac, M.D.
Director, de L'Unite Recherches,
Inserm,
Bordeaux, France

E. Thoreson, M.D.
Hôpital Pellegrin,
Service des Isotopes,
Place Amelie Raba-Leon,
Bordeaux, France

In its present state, ocular scintigraphy permits only a relatively small percentage of ocular tumors to be detected (melanomas) because of the utilization of specific radioactive vectors for this type of tumor.[1] Metastases and other primitive tumors cannot be detected by this method of investigation. Phosphorus-32 cannot be employed for the external detection of posterior tumors because of the weak penetration power of β particles. In order to get around this disadvantage, we have utilized the Cerenkov effect produced by β particles from ^{32}P in vitreous tumors.[2] This allows the detection of the concentration of this isotope in the posterior half of the eye.

TECHNOLOGY

In the medical application, the range of detection is composed of the Cerenkov effect detector, an optical apparatus that collects light produced in this detector, and the electronic apparatus associated with it.

The detector of the Cerenkov effect is the eye itself. The β^- particles emitted by ^{32}P which is fixed in the tumor, in crossing the vitreous tumor produces light when their energy is above 0.264 MeV. The spectral range of this light takes place in the ultraviolet and in the visible light range.[3] Because of the directing feature of the Cerenkov effect, the light is directed anteriorly and focused through by the pupil. The crystalline lens becomes a filter and a lens. At 380 nm, the ultraviolet light produces a fluorescence of the crystalline lens owing to the activation of electrons of two crystalline components: lactoflavine and alloxazine.[4] Because of this fluorescence, it is impossible to detect exactly where the tumor is located.

The light, therefore, is transmitted from the eye using an intermediary optic guide (light pipe) to the photocathode of a photomultiplier. The photomultiplier (5G DUVP RTC) was chosen for its high sensitivity in the spectral region where the Cerenkov effect is important. We have ameliorated the performance of this tube by using a cooling system (at +5°C) and a system of thermal isolation. If too much cooling is applied, however, the sensitivity of the tube is diminished. Between the photocathode and the light pipe is an obturator, which permits the stabilization of background current. Thus the detected signal is adapted, amplified, and analyzed by an amplitude selector.

PROCEDURE

The results of the first experiments have allowed us to improve the detection of the Cerenkov effect before its application in the human eye.

First Experiment: Detection of the Cerenkov Effect in the Normal Eye of a Rabbit (Fig. 1)

An intravenous injection of 1 mCi of ^{32}P was given to a rabbit 24 hours before enucleation. The count of the Cerenkov signal and that of background noise lasted for 10 minutes and for 100 minutes, respectively. These first experiments were done without the light pipe. It is believed that the analyzed signal is not only the Cerenkov effect produced in the eye but also the one that is produced in the photocathode. This problem is eliminated with the utilization of a light pipe (Fig. 2). Results of one preliminary experiment are summarized in Figs. 3, 4, and 5.

96

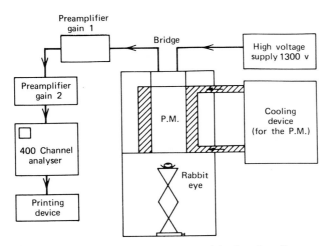

Fig. 1.   Schematic diagram of the apparatus used for detection of the Cerenkov effect.

A low concentration of phosphorus is found in cornea, crystalline lens, and vitreous humour. A high concentration of phosphorus is found in iris, ciliary body, choroid, retina, and muscles of the eye. Because of these concentrations, we can detect Cerenkov light in the eye. In turning the posterior half of the eye toward the photocathode, we find that the signal is inferior to the one produced when the anterior half is posed in front of the photocathode.

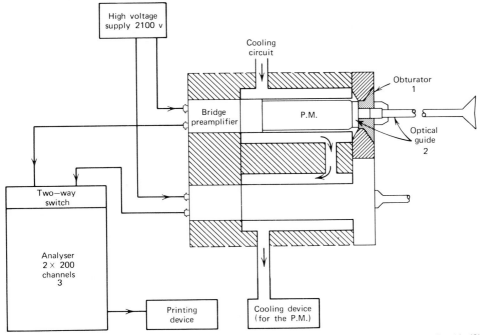

Fig. 2.   Same apparatus as previously in its principle but equipped with an obturator (1), an optical guide (2) to transmit the light from the eye, and analyzer (3) using twice 200 channels.

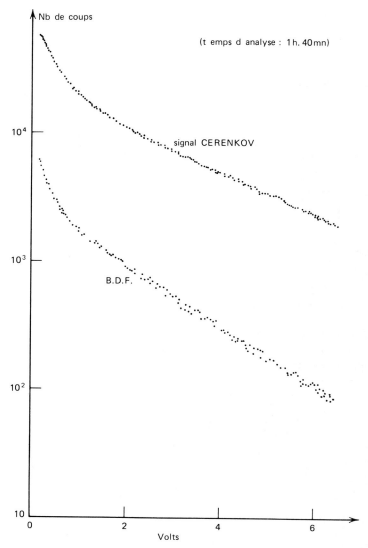

Fig. 3. Curves obtained for background and Cerenkov signal—(number of counts voltage of the analyzer). Counting time: 100 minutes.

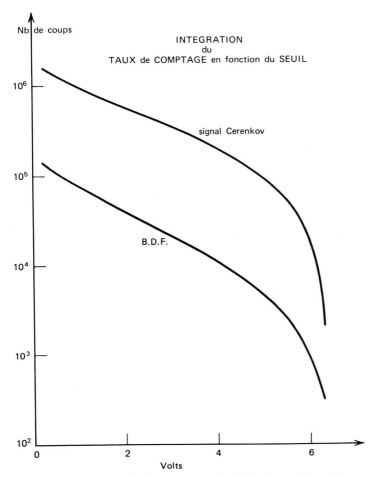

Fig. 4.   Integrated number of counts versus threshold voltage of the analyzer.

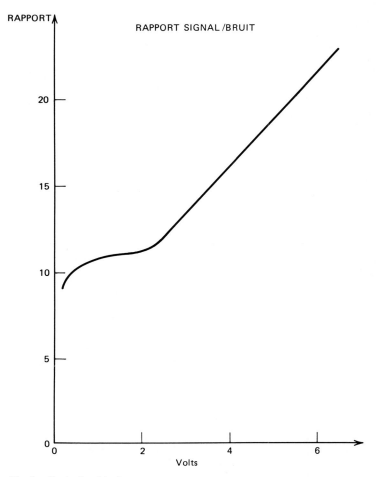

Fig. 5. Ratio signal/noise.

TABLE 1

Background	Time	Count[a]	Count Rate[a] (cpm)
Noise	2.000 s	8.799	264
Eye placed 4 cm from photocathode	2.000 s	21.016	630
Lens between eye and photocathode	2.000 s	16.540	496
Black sheet of paper between eye and photo- cathode	2.000 s	14.578	437

[a] Numbers indicated are averages.

Second Experiment: A Global Analysis of the Signal

To understand exactly what this signal was, we carried out several experiments. In one experiment we put a lens between the photocathode and the eye. In the other one, we put a black sheet of paper between the photocathode and the eye (see Table 1).

CONCLUSION

Before actually passing on to the detection of tumor of human eyes, we must statistically evaluate the validity of this method in rabbits. A graft of tumor cells, must be applied from a *"green strain"* to the eye of a rabbit. The comparison must then be made between a normal eye and one with a tumor.

REFERENCES

1. Safi, N.: Apports des Molécules Marquées dans l'Étude des Tumeurs Mélaniques Expérimentales et Humaines. Thèse doctorat d'etat en biologie humaine, 1974.
2. Burch, W. H.: Cerenkov light from ^{32}P as an Aid to Diagnosis of Eye Tumour. *Nature* 234:358 (1971).
3. Frank, I. M., and Tamm, I.: Coherent Visible Radiation of Fast Electrons Passing Through Matter. *Dokl. Akad. Nauk. S.S.S.R* 14 (3):109 (1937).
4. Greenfield, M. A., Norman, A., Dowdy, A. H., and Kratz, P. M.: β and γ Induced Cerenkov Radiation in Water. *J. Opt. Soc. Am.* 43 (1):42 (1953).
5. Saraux, H., and Biais, B.: Physiologie oculaire. *Masson Editeur,* Paris, 1973.
6. Charman, W. N., Dennis, J. A., Fazio, G. G., and Jelley, S. V.: Visual Sensations Produced by Single Fast Particles. *Nature* 230:522–524 (1971).
7. Fazio, G. G., Jelley, J. V., and Charman, W. N.: Generation by Cerenkov Light Flashes by Cosmic Radiation Within the Eyes of the Apollo Astronauts. *Nature* 228:260–264 (1970).
8. Jelley, J. V.: *Cerenkov Radiation and Its Applications.* Pergamon Press, London, 1958.

The Chemistry of Radiopharmaceuticals for Noncontact Detection of Ocular Tumors

Ned D. Heindel, Ph.D.
Professor of Chemistry,
Lehigh University;
Associate Professor,
Department of Radiation Therapy,
and Nuclear Medicine
Hahnemann Medical College,
Philadelphia, Pennsylvania

One of the major thrusts of nuclear medicine research in recent years has been the development of specific tumor-localizing radiopharmaceuticals for key organs.[1] The problems with the diagnostic accuracy[7] of the traditional ^{32}P test for ocular melanoma have spawned research studies into more than a score of candidate radiopharmaceuticals, not only for delineation of this neoplasm but also for other tumors of the orbit and globe. Furthermore, the manipulatory difficulties[10] involved in the contact detection required for the weakly penetrating beta-emitters, such as ^{32}P, have caused radiopharmaceutical researchers to focus on the gamma-emitting isotopes which are more useful for external imaging with rectilinear scanners and gamma cameras. As is so often the case in an evolving science such as diagnostic nuclear medicine, the empirical fact-gathering process must proceed in the absence of a comprehensive underlying theoretical base. Thus, those common chemical features, if indeed such features do exist, which facilitate the incorporation of chemical compounds into ocular neoplasms are presently unknown. We cannot yet plan new tumor-localizing compounds from a purely theoretical viewpoint.

From a physical viewpoint, however, it is possible to cite three concepts that operate to explain the localization of the successful tumor-detecting radiopharmaceuticals: (1) an increased permeability of the capillaries in tumors for any chemical substance (often referred to as the concept of "hypervascularity" or "abnormal permeability"); (2) an abnormally high demand by the tumor for the components and precursors of cellular metabolism such as phosphate, nucleotides, nucleosides, peptides, and amino acids (often referred to as the concept of "differential kinetics"); and (3) the existence of specific complexation or bonding of a radiotagged agent within the neoplastic tissue. The latter line might include the studies on labeled antineoplastic agents and on labeled antibodies which are specific for tumor components as delineating probes for malignancies. This review summarizes the various chemical entities that have been evaluated as ocular radiopharmaceuticals and attempts to convey the underlying rationale that prompted their synthesis.

AGENTS FUNCTIONING BY HYPERVASCULARITY OF TUMORS

In the early 1960s, several groups utilizing blood-pool agents and relying on the hypervacularity of intraocular neoplasms investigated ^{131}I-human serum albumin[2,3] and radioiodinated derivatives of the classic agent for ophthalmic angiography, fluorescein.[4] In a study involving 17 patients with ^{125}I-diiodofluorescein, Goren, Newell, Brizel, and Harper determined that eyes harboring neoplasms invariably incorporated the isotope to a 23% excess compared to control eyes when measured after 8 hours postdosing.[4] Although the patient grouping studied was small, there were no false-positives and only one false-negative, a patient with a metastatic adenocarcinoma of the choroid.

A later report by Newell evaluating ^{125}I-diiodofluorescein by a similar protocol (20% difference between counts in tumor-bearing and control eyes taken at 8 hours postinjection of 5 μCi/kg dose of the agent) claimed a diagnostic accuracy of 73%.[5] The 22 patients involved in this study possessed histologically confirmed intraocular and intraorbital lesions, and with the 20% difference criterion there were no false-positives and six false-negatives. Blanquet recently reported on the use of ^{131}I-diiodofluorescein as a probe for the hypervascularity associated with ocular tumors but concluded that ^{99m}Tc pertechnetate was more advantageous.[6] Similarly, Beierwaltes[7] in general comments on iodofluorescein as a tumor-detecting radiopharmaceutical cited studies[8] which found an unacceptably high number of false-negative results.

[131]I-human serum albumin has long been known to be a blood-pool agent and to be in equilibrium with ocular blood in an equilibrium favored by administration of vasodilators.[2] However, studies of its ability to localize melanomas in hamsters were unsuccessful,[9] and only 25% of malignant human ocular tumors gave positive results in a recent Yugoslavian clinical study.[3] The radiopharmaceutical was, however, very successful in delineating orbital angiomas and benign tumors, especially when these were located in the superior temporal portion of the orbit.[3]

In a related vein, [197]Hg-chlormerodrin, which binds rapidly and nearly quantitatively (85%) to plasma proteins[11] and hence has been exploited as a brain-scanning agent, has also been studied in ocular neoplasms. Sodee[12] was one of the first investigators to claim the utility of radio-chlormerodrin, bearing the [203]Hg isotope, in ocular tumor detection, but no statistical data were given to judge the reliability of the method. In a study of 59 patients with unilateral exophthalmos, 24 tumors of various types were delineated by scanning but 4 pseudotumors were also read as neoplasms and 1 malignancy was missed with [197]Hg-chlormerodrin.[13]

A more extensive investigation involving 134 patents was reported, again all characterized by unilateral exophthalmos. Scanning was performed at 2½ hours postdosing with 20 μCi/kg of [197]Hg-chlormerodrin and the orbits were viewed anteriorly with the chin depressed to lengthen the exposure to the detector. Lateral radioactivity was also mapped by scanning the entire orbit and the adjacent intracranial areas. A marked asymmetry of isotope distribution, according to a quantified scale of four gradations, was taken as indication of a malignancy. Seven of the 52 known tumors produced negative scans, and 16 pseudotumors (mostly orbital granulomas) were read as malignancies. In accord with results obtained in hamster melanomas by Beierwaltes and co-workers in which no specific uptake of the [197]Hg-chlormerodrin by the melanin-containing tissues was observed, the clinical investigations also did not demonstrate any selectivity of the radiopharmaceutical toward delineation of ocular melanomas.[14]

Sodium pertechnetate-^{99m}Tc, long established as a blood-pool imaging agent useful in detecting brain tumors, has been similarly evaluated as a localizer of orbital neoplasms. Trokel's group found it less preferable than [197]Hg-chlormerodin because the peak period for maximum uptake of the [99m]TcO$_4^-$ into orbital tissues occurred at shorter times postdosing and took place over a narrower time span.[14] Thus, a more critical time for imaging was required with the technetium nuclide as opposed to the mercury one. However, the superior physical and dosimetric characteristics of ^{99m}Tc and the improved quality of the images obtained, especially with use of an Anger camera, pinhole collimator, and computerized multiparametric analysis system, led Blanquet to favor pertechnetate over the other radiopharmaceuticals which function as probes of hypervascularization.[6] Since high background uptake of sodium pertechnetate in the tissues surrounding the orbital region is very commonly observed, the utilization of an electronic color enhancement program to increase orbital detail was found greatly to facilitate scan interpretation.[15] This method, applied to the study of 33 patients with orbital disease, correctly localized the intraorbital mass with respect to the globe in 13 out of the 14 patient cases deemed to display positive scans. Using a combination of a comparative count method in a 21-patient study to indicate differential uptake and a scanning follow-up to pinpoint the area of enhanced radioactivity in a 21-patient study, Heuer and Ehler found sodium pertechnetate useful in localizing the proliferative tissue. As expected for agents which operate by hypervascularization uptake, the radiopharmaceutical could not distinguish malignancies from pseudotumors.[16]

The much-studied radiopharmaceutical for tumor imaging, ^{67}Ga-citrate, has also been investigated in tumors of the orbit and globe. Mori, Hamamoto, and Torizuka,[17] without indicating the specific tumor type, have reported that ^{67}Ga-citrate successfully localized tumors as small as 1.5 cm in diameter. However, they also observed numerous false-positives due to uptake in inflammatory and granulomatous sites. Heuer and co-workers[18] have stated firmly that ^{67}Ga-citrate is not useful in detecting malignant melanoma of the choroid, for in only one of nine confirmed cases was hyperactivity observed in the malignancy. A selectivity for tumor uptake by ^{67}Ga-citrate would not be expected in light of the numerous nonmalignant situations in which functioning glandular tissue,[19] abscesses,[20] infarcts,[21] and other inflammatory conditions[22] concentrate the nuclide, but the high percentage of false-negatives reported by Heuer is somewhat unexpected.

AGENTS FUNCTIONING BY DIFFERENTIAL KINETICS OF METABOLISM

The second of the major rationales employed to explain radiopharmaceutical incorporation by a tumor is the higher than normal demand by the tumor for the components and precursors of cellular metabolism. The ^{32}P-phosphate uptake can be explained on these grounds, and similar reasoning has been employed in the synthesis and evaluation of many other candidate radiopharmaceuticals for the eye.

Taking a clue from numerous biochemical studies on inhibition of DNA synthesis by the selective and competitive antagonist of thymidine, 5-iodo-2′-desoxyuridine,[23] Filippone synthesized the radio-labeled counterpart, ^{125}I-5-iodo-2′-desoxyuridine.[24] In preclinical studies in rabbits whose sclera had been inoculated with transplant fragments of the Brown-Pearce tumor, the radiopharmaceutical was claimed to successfully localize the areas of malignant growth.

In a purely basic science study, Miura measured the uptake kinetics and ocular distribution of a vitamin B_1 derivative, thiamine propyl disulfide-[35]S.[25] This derivative is known to possess biochemistry similar to thiamine itself but to be more rapidly absorbed than the parent agent.[26] By utilization of a microautoradiographic method applied to rabbit eyes, the radiopharmaceutical was found to concentrate in uvea and optic nerve tissue to a much greater extent than in vitreous and lens. No application of the agent as a candidate tumor-localizing radiopharmaceutical was reported.

Similarly, chemical agents known to exert a pharmacologic action upon some element within the eye might, at some future date, be developed into useful diagnostic radiopharmaceuticals for ocular malignancies. Kramer and Potts established that the iris avidly extracts exogenous catecholamines (such as norepinephrine) from the blood[27] and the uptake and distribution of a tritiated analog were measured. A pro-drug form of epinephrine with its hydroxyls esterified with lipophilic carboxylates has been reported to be absorbed much more rapidly than epinephrine itself but no tissue distribution was reported.[28] Often employed for inflammatory and allergic conditions of the eye, hydrocortisone has been radio-labeled with ^{3}H and ^{14}C and its absorption pathway following subconjunctival injection (diffusion from sclera through choroid to retina) has been monitored.[29, 30] Reasoning that the lower native concentration of urea in the aqueous humor, compared to plasma, might represent a selective exclusion of this agent, Goren and Newell investigated the uptake of ^{14}C urea in rabbit eyes. The ^{14}C urea, administered by IV injection and monitored by autoradiographic imaging of the enucleated eyes at 2 hours postdosing, was indeed found in the outer tissues of the eye with the anterior surfaces of the iris and ciliary process receiving the highest dose.[31] Whether any of these observations will lead to useful ocular radiopharmaceuticals depends largely on the distribution of the candidate agent within tumor-bearing eyes; these experiments have not been done.

AGENTS FUNCTIONING BY SPECIFIC COMPLEXATION OR BONDING

The third of the major rationales utilized to explain radiopharmaceutical uptake by an ocular tumor is the existence of a specific complexation or specific bonding of the radiolabeled agent within the neoplastic tissue. This "binding" must occur to a significantly greater extent within the tumor than in the surrounding benign tissue. The concept of employing labeled antitumor agents as probes for tumor localization has been reviewed elsewhere,[1] but it should be noted here that chelates of the anticancer antibiotic bleomycin are currently showing the greatest promise in clinical applications. A preliminary report on the ^{99m}Tc complex of bleomycin for imaging tumors of the orbit was encouraging, but specific details of the types of tumors delineated has not yet been provided.[17] The striking therapeutic success reported in the treatment of intraocular melanoma with the nitroso urea agent BCNU[32] might point to the possible success of a labeled analog of this drug as a melanoma-detecting radiopharmaceutical.

Certainly the most successful melanoma-delineating agents are the radio-iodinated chloroquine analogs. The clinical experience with this class has been discussed by other authors in this volume but the chemistry of the agents and mechanism of their localiza-

Chloroquine

Labeling and final structure of Beierwaltes' NM-113.

Blanquet's radio-iodinated chloroquine derivative.

tion are best treated in this chapter. From strict chemical nomenclature rules, "iodo-chloroquine" is a misnomer, for it does not precisely define a single chemical entity, and furthermore at least two different radiopharmaceuticals loosely defined as "iodo-chloroquine" have been considered. Initial feasibility studies with a ^{14}C-labeled chloroquine, correctly named 4-(4-diethylamino-1-methylbutylamino)-7-chloro-quinoline, showed excellent uptake in hamster melanomas.[9] These studies led to the synthesis of a radio-iodinated derivative[33] prepared by thermally induced nucleophilic displacement by ^{125}I of the #7 chloro in 4-(3-dimethylaminopropylamino)-7-chloro-quinoline. The resulting radiopharmaceutical, designated as NM-113, has received the most intense animal and clinical scrutiny.[34] Much of the work in Blanquet's laboratory has been carried out on an electrophilically radio-iodinated chloroquine which represents yet a third member of this family, 4-(4-diethylamino-1-methylbutylamino)-6-iodo-7-chloroquinoline.

An explanation for the melanophilia of these chloroquine analogs must take cognizance of the historical background on the therapeutic effects of aminoquinolines and of the deductive reasoning which led to their initial evaluation as ocular radiopharmaceuticals. Long known to induce ocular opacities and other unpleasant visual side effects as a consequence of chronic high dosage therapy, chloroquine, chlorpromazine, and other benzo-fused heterocyclic drugs were shown by Potts to display an active affinity for melanin.[35, 36] The molecular origin of this affinity rests in the formation of a charge transfer complex between the electron-rich heterocyclic drug—which is chloroquine in the case being considered herein—and the electron-poor, highly oxidized melanin.[37] The biosynthesis of melanin from tyrosine, substantial portions of which have been duplicated in vitro, represents a complex series of oxidative one electron losses.[38] The replicating melanoprotein extracts an electron from the chloroquine-melanin charge transfer complex, leaving behind a chloroquine free radical.[37] There is additional evidence to suggest that the newly formed free radical intercalates between the strands of DNA in the protein portion of the melanoprotein.[39] Chloroquine itself not only intercalates DNA but is also held rigidly in position by a specific electrostatic interaction between the 2-amino group of guanine and the electronegative 7-halo atom of the chloroquine moiety.[40] Interactions such as these are presumably responsible for the impressive melanophilia of the iodinated chloroquine radiopharmaceuticals.

The recent substantial increase in cooperative programs in nuclear medicine research in which biochemists, medicinal chemists, physiologists, and clinicians direct their joint efforts at improved tumor and organ imaging agents, will undoubtedly produce a new generation of noncontact ocular radiopharmaceuticals. The three theoretical bases of hypervascularity, differential kinetics and specific intratumor bonding can provide a useful foundation for new research in ocular tumor imaging agents, but substantial consideration will also have to be paid to the biochemistry and physiology of the eye in the design and evaluation of new candidate diagnostics.

REFERENCES

1. Heindel, N. D.: The Chemical Foundation of Tumor Localization. In Croll, M., Brady, L. W., Honda, T., and Wallner, R. J., Eds., *New Techniques in Tumor Localization and Radioimmunoassay*, John Wiley, New York, 1974, pp. 83–92.

2. Fukushi, S.: Measurement of Ocular Blood Volume by Injection of ^{131}I-Albumin in Rabbits. *Acta Soc. Ophthalmol. Japan* **66**:335–339 (1962).

3. Litricin, O., Pendie, S., Ilic, R., and Nlagojevic, M.: Gamma Orbitography. *Ann. Ocul.* **204**:1317–1330 (1971).

4. Goren, S. B., Newell, F. W., Brizel, H. E., and Harper, P. V.: The Use of I-125 Labelled Di-iodo-fluorescein. *Am. J. Ophthalmol.* **54**:191–196 (1962).

5. Newell, F. W.: Iodine-125 Labeled Diiodofluorescein in the Diagnosis of Intraocular Tumors. *J. Nucl. Med.* **5**:314–315 (1964).

6. Blanquet, P., Verin, P., Basse-Cathalinat, B., and Safi, N.: Ocular Scintigraphy. *J. Nucl. Med.* **15**:478 (1974).

7. Boyd, C. M., Beierwaltes, W. H., Lieberman, L. M., and Bergstrom, T. J.: ^{125}I-Labeled Chloroquine Analogs in Diagnosis of Ocular Melanomas. *J. Nucl. Med.* **12**:601–605 (1971).

8. Leopold, I. H.: Role of Isotopes in Diagnosis of Intraocular Neoplasms. *Trans. Am. Opthalmol. Soc.* **62**:86–99 (1964).

9. Beierwaltes, W. H., Varma, V. M., Lieberman, L. M., Counsell, R. E., and Morales, J.: Scintillation Scanning of Malignant Melanomas with Radioiodinated Quinoline Derivatives. *J. Lab. Clin. Med.* **72**:485–494 (1968).

10. Carmichael, P. L., Holst, G. C., Federman, J. L., Shields, J. A.: The Present Status of the [32]P Test in Ophthalmology. In Croll, M., Brady, L. W., Honda, T., and Wallner, R. J., Eds., *New Techniques in Tumor Localization and Radioimmunoassay*, John Wiley, New York, 1974, pp. 193–202.

11. Soloway, A. H., and Davis, M. A.: Survey of Radiopharmaceuticals and Their Current Status. *J. Pharm. Sci.* **63**:654 (1974).

12. Sodee, D. B.: Localization of Eye Tumor by External Counting with [203]Hg-Neohydrin. *J. Nucl. Med.* **4**:194 (1963).

13. Schlesinger, E. B., Trokel, S. L., and Bailey, S.: Radioactive Scanning in the Analysis of Unilateral Exophthalmos. *Trans. Am. Acad. Ophthalmol. Otolaryng.* **73**:1005–1012 (1969).

14. Trokel, S. L., Schlesinger, E. B., and Beaton, H.: Diagnosis of Orbital Tumors by Gamma-Ray Orbitography. *Am. J. Ophthalmol.* **74**:675–679 (1972).

15. Kramer, S. G., Archer, D. D., Polcyn, R. E., Charleston, D. B., and Yasillo, N.: Color Enhancement of Brain and Orbital Scans in Proptosis. *Trans. Am. Acad. Ophthalmol. Otolaryng.* **74**:1240–1248 (1970).

16. Heuer, H. E., and Ehlers, N.: Orbitography with Technetium 99m for Evaluation of Orbital Tumors. *Ann. Ocul.* **205**:283–290 (1972).

17. Mori, T., Hamamoto, K., and Torizuka, K.: Studies on the Usefulness of ^{99m}Tc-Labeled Bleomycin for Tumor Imaging. *J. Nucl. Med.* **14**:431 (1973).

18. Heuer, H. E., Ehlers, N., and Hansen, H. H.: Malignant Melanoma of the Choroid. *Ann. Ocul.* **205**:1109–1113 (1972).

19. Mishkin, F. S., and Maynard, W. P.: Lacrimal Gland Accumulation of [67]Ga. *J. Nucl. Med.* **15**:630–631 (1974).

20. Fratkin, M. J., Hirsch, J. I., and Sharpe, A. R.: Ga-67 Localization of Post-Operative Abdominal Abscesses. *J. Nucl. Med.* **15**:491 (1974).

21. Zweiman, F. G., O'Keefe, A., Idoine, J., Camin, L. L., and Holman, B. L.: Selectivity of Uptake by ^{99m}Tc-Chelates and ^{67}Ga in Acutely Infarcted Myocardium. *J. Nucl. Med.* **15**:546–547 (1974).

22. Waxman, A. D., and Siemsen, J. K.: Gallium Scanning of the Gall Bladder. *J. Nucl. Med.* **15**:543 (1974).

23. Welch, A. D.: 5-Iodo-2′-Deoxyuridine and Its Analogs. In Kimura, S. J., and Goodner, E. K., Eds., *Ocular Pharmacology and Therapeutics*, F. A. Davis, Philadelphia, 1964, pp. 197–214.

24. Filippone, C. C.: ^{125}I-Desoxyuridine. *G. Ital. Oftal.* **16**:392–395 (1963).

25. Miura, S.: The Uptake and Distribution of Thiamine Propyl Disulfide ^{35}S in Rabbit Eyes. *Acta Soc. Ophthalmol. Japan* **69**:792–808 (1965).

26. Matsukawa, F.: Thiamine Propyl Disulfide. *J. Vitaminol.* **1**:13 (1954); and *The Merck Index*, 8th Ed., Merck and Co., Rahway, N.J., 1968, p. 1037.

27. Kramer, S. G., and Potts, A. M.: Iris Uptake of Cathecholamines in Experimental Horner's Syndrome. *Am. J. Ophthalmol.* **67**:705–713 (1969).

28. Ackerman, B., Buddrus, D. J., Eriksen, S., and McClure, D. A.: The Influence of a Pro-Drug Route on the Administration of Epinephrine. Abstracts of Medicinal Chemistry, 168th Am. Chem. Soc. Meeting, 1974, Number 23.

29. Wine, N. A., Gornall, A. G., and Basu, P. K.: The Ocular Uptake of Subconjunctivally Injected ^{14}C-Hydrocortisone. *Am. J. Ophthalmol.* **58**:362–366 (1964).

30. Drysdale, I. O., Gornall, A. G., Kiseilins, D., and Basu, P. K.: The Ocular Uptake of ^{3}H-Hydrocortisone. *Am. J. Ophthalmol.* **56**:838 (1961).

31. Goren, S. B., and Newell, F. W.: The Autoradiographic Localization of Urea-^{14}C in the Rabbit Eye. *Am. J. Ophthalmol.* **54**:63–66 (1962).

32. Stark, W. J. Jr., Rosenthal, A. R., Mullins, G. M., and Greem, W. R.: Simultaneous Bilateral Uveal Melanomas Responding to BCNU Therapy. *Trans. Am. Acad. Ophthalmol. Otolaryng.* **75**:70–83 (1971).

33. Counsell, R. E., Pocha, P., Morales, J. O., and Beierwaltes, W. H.: Tumor Localizing Agents: III. Radioiodinated Quinoline Derivatives. *J. Pharm. Sci.* **56**:1042–1044 (1967).

34. Beierwaltes, W. H.: Labeled Chloroquine Analog in Diagnosis of Ocular and Dermal Melanomas. In Croll, M., Brady, L. W., Honda, T., and Wallner, R. J., Ed., *New Techniques in Tumor Localization and Radioimmunoassay,* John Wiley, New York, 1974, pp. 161–171.

35. Potts, A. M.: The Concentration of Phenothiazines in the Eye of Experimental Animals. *Invest. Ophthalmol.* **1**:522–530 (1962).

36. Potts, A. M.: The Reactions of Uveal Pigment In Vitro with Polycyclic Compounds. *Invest. Ophthalmol.* **3**:399–417 (1964).

37. Carr, C. J.: Melanin Affinity and Psychopharmacologic Effects of Drugs. *Psychopharmacol. Bull.* **10**(4):38–40 (October 1974).

38. Young, T. E., Griswold, J. R., and Hulbert, M. H.: Melanin. I. Kinetics of the Oxidative Cyclization of Dopa to Dopachrome. *J. Org. Chem.* **39**:1980–1982 (1974).

39. Ohnishi, S., and McConnell, H. M.: Interaction of the Radical Ion of Chlorpromazine with Deoxyribonucleic Acid. *J. Am. Chem. Soc.* **87**:2293 (1965).

40. Although the intercalation experiments (see following reference) were carried out on chloroquine, the free radical evidence was collected on chlorpromazine. Since the chemical structures and the respective melanophilias of these agents are similar, it is probable that their mechanisms of localization are similar. See Hahn, F. E., O'Brien, R. L., Ciak, J., Allison, J. L., and Olenick, J. G.: Studies on the Modes of Action of Chloroquine, Quinacrine, and Quinine and on Chloroquine Resistance. *Military Med.,* Special Supplement, pp. 1071–1089 (1966).

Short-Lived Radiopharmaceuticals for Noncontact Detection of Ocular Melanoma

Samuel Packer, M.D.
Clinical Instructor,
Department of Ophthalmology,
Cornell University School of Medicine,
Manhattan, New York

R. M. Lambrecht, Ph.D.
Chemist,
Brookhaven National Laboratory,
Upton, Long Island, New York

H. L. Atkins, M.D.
Senior Scientist, Medical Department,
Brookhaven National Laboratory,
Upton, Long Island, New York

A. P. Wolf, Ph.D.
Senior Scientist of Chemistry,
Brookhaven National Laboratory,
Upton, Long Island, New York

A major advantage in the use of radionuclides with short physical half-lives in nuclear ophthalmology is the low radiation dose to the lens. This is particularly important with a compound that selectively localizes in an ocular melanoma and has a long biological half-life. The use of short-lived radiopharmaceuticals with reduced radiation exposure from each procedure permits the studies to be repeated, and suspicious lesions can be followed. By selecting the appropriate radionuclide, an adequate photon energy level can be obtained (50–300 keV) that will have adequate tissue penetration and allow the use of noninvasive techniques.[1] Patients with lesions which were not obviously malignant melanomas would be more readily evaluated, as would patients with opaque media. The half-life of the radionuclide cannot be too short because time must elapse before the differential uptake between tumor and background tissues is large enough to allow detection.

The ratio between uptake of the radiopharmaceutical by a tumor versus background will reach a maximum after a certain time has elapsed. The time course will determine the appropriate half-life and determine when detection of a tumor in a given organ is possible. Wagner and Emmons[2] state that the ideal radiopharmaceutical should have an optimum physical half-life equal to $1n2 \times$ the time of the observation. Thus the biological behavior must be ascertained. The bond between the tumor-seeking agent and the radioisotope must be stable in vivo, and the ideal compound would be one that is tumor specific. Radio-labeled immune substances which are tumor associated have been used clinically, but have quantitative limitations. The number of available receptor sites for these compounds is crucial if it is to be detectable. However, the high degree of specificity would be a favorable factor.[3] At present, we are concerned with agents of only relative value in tumor localization; therefore, factors such as biological behavior and performance of detection devices become very important.

Preclinical evaluation of radiopharmaceuticals with an animal model and a phantom permits screening of compounds and comparison of the relative value of various agents. In addition, the problem of background can be delineated, determining whether the agents also go to choroid, retina, bone, blood, muscle, and other organs. By looking at the time course of radioactivity in the tumor relative to other tissues, we can determine the optimum time for detection.

Several categories of compounds can be used as tumor-localizing agents. Blanquet and Safi[4] have reviewed the development of radiopharmaceuticals for use in nuclear ophthalmology to 1974. Of these we have concentrated on the development of new nuclides and labeled compounds with suspected pigment affinity, for example, iodinated chloroquine analogs (^{123}I-4,3 DMQ), heavy metals (lead-203 and thallium-201), antibiotics (^{57}Co-bleomycin), and metabolites (^{32}P). Our results obtained with ^{123}I-4,3-DMQ [i.e., 4-(3-dimethylaminopropylamino)-7-iodoquinoline] are the topic of another paper.[5] This chapter focuses attention on our recent work with an inorganic coordination compound of ^{203}Pb.

Lead-203 seems to offer several advantages as a potential radionuclide in radiopharmaceutical applications. Certain heavy metals localize in tumors.[6, 7, 8] There is additional evidence that heavy metals have an affinity for melanin.[9] However, localization of metals in tumors is not a constant finding.[10, 11] We are searching for a chemical form of lead-203 that is appropriate for localization in malignant melanoma.

Research carried out at BNL under contract with the U.S. Energy Research and Development Administration. This research supported in part by grant CA16316 from the National Cancer Institutes.

112

The physical characteristics of ^{203}Pb are suitable for scintigraphy with available equipment.[12] It decays with a 52.1 hour half-life by electron capture with the emission of 279 keV photons in 95% abundance. The half-life of ^{203}Pb allows for its shipment to medical centers that do not have a cyclotron available. The half-life also allows for biological time to elapse, permitting background concentration to decrease while tumor concentration stabilizes, and favors tumor detection.

METHODS

Carrier-free ^{203}Pb was produced on the BNL 60′ cyclotron using the ^{203}Tl(d,2n) → ^{203}Pb nuclear reaction with the deuterons degraded from 22.7 → 0 MeV in a target of 99.99% purity thallium metal. The chemical separation of the ^{203}Pb from the target resulted in a radiochemical purity in excess of 99.99%.[12] Lead-203-tris was prepared by addition of an aqueous solution of 2-amino-2-hydroxymethyl,1,3-propanediol to the carrier-free ^{203}Pb.[8] The ligand is also known as tris, or tromethamine, and is commonly used in tris and Tham biological buffer. The solution was adjusted to pH 6.8–7.2. Passage through a millipore filter assured sterility of the labeled compound after its preparation. Details of the design of the radiopharmaceutical are found elsewhere.[3, 15] Additional radiopharmaceuticals tested were ^{57}Co-bleomycin and thallium-201 chloride.*

The Greene melanoma in the male Syrian golden hamster was used as the experimental model.[13] Skin tumors are transplanted every 2 weeks. This time is optimal for testing since there is minimal necrosis and tumor size is adequate for biopsy. For ocular tumors, a cell suspension was made from 1.0 g of skin melanoma which was cut into small pieces, mixed with 5.0 ml of a tissue culture medium, and forced through a microsieve (27 μ pores). This resulted in approximately 50 cells per microliter with a moderate amount of cell clumping. Cell viability as determined with the trypan blue stain was approximately 75–80%. Animals were anesthetized with ether. With the aid of an operating microscope (25×) the globe was rotated and held firmly with a small muscle hook. A straight pin was used to penetrate conjunctiva and sclera. Swirling the pen against a firm globe permitted a track to be made through the sclera while avoiding uncontrolled puncture of the globe and entry in the vitreous cavity. A 30-gauge needle was inserted into the track and passed posteriorly beneath the sclera for a short distance. A definite attempt was made to have the injection intrachoroidal. After 5.0 μl of the cell suspension was injected, Eastman 910 glue was placed over the injection site while the needle was still in the eye. The glue was given time to harden slightly *and* the needle withdrawn. Antibiotic ointment was applied at the end of the procedure.

Dissections were done after 2 to 3 weeks of tumor growth. Various organs were taken from hamsters either skin or eye melanoma. Detailed dissection of the various parts of the eye was done with the aid of the operating microscope. Large specimens such as liver or kidney were placed in larger vials. Small specimens, such as, cornea, retina, and so forth, were placed in gelatin capsules and then into small vials. Because of the light weight of the individual detailed parts of the eye, each gelatin capsule contained four specimens. All vials, with or without gelatin capsules, were preweighed. After all tissues were in the vials, they were reweighed to give tissue weights. The radioactivity was assayed on an automatic gamma counter.† The data was corrected for radioactive decay

---

* The ^{57}Co-bleomycin was provided by Dr. W. C. Eckelman, Department of Nuclear Medicine, Washington Hospital Center, Washington, D.C. Thallium-201 is available from New England Nuclear Corp.
† Nuclear-Chicago, Des Plaines, Illinois, Model 1185.

and the like and calculated as the percent uptake per gram of tissue relative to the total injected dose.

RESULTS

Table 1 has the percent uptake for lead-203-tris by the skin and eye melanoma, parts of the eye, and the various organs of the hamster. Figure 1 shows that the kidney, liver, and bone have a substantial uptake. The uptake in eye melanoma peaks at 24 hours, while the skin melanoma reaches maximum uptake at 6 hours.

The amount of uptake by background tissues is important if one is considering scintigraphy. Therefore, an inspection of the uptake by other ocular tissues reveals that the primary competitor is the choroid. Figure 2 shows that the greatest ratio between ocular tumor and choroid (i.e., ~ 3.6) occurs at 24 hours. The ratio of percent uptake per gram of tumor eye to the normal eye was $\sim 25:1$. The obvious implication is that ocular tumor scanning or counting with a collimated probe should be done at this time. However, the in vivo problem is much more complex and background consists also of orbital bone, blood, brain, muscle, and so forth (Table 1). For certain organs with high uptake, such as the liver and kidney, it is doubtful from results with this tumor model

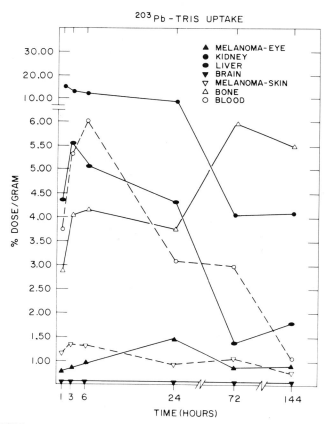

Fig. 1.   Uptake of ^{203}Pb-tris in various organs of the hamster at 1 to 144 hours.

TABLE 1. DISTRIBUTION OF CARRIER-FREE LEAD-203 TRIS IN PERCENT UPTAKE PER GRAM OF TISSUE AT VARIOUS TIMES[a]

Tissue	Time					
	1	3	6	24	72	144
Melanoma-eye	1.048 ±0.214	0.976 ±0.190	1.609 ±0.306	1.314 ±0.188	0.724* ±0.260	0.821 ±0.150
Normal-eye	0.200 ±0.037	0.086 ±0.010	0.111 ±0.011	0.054 ±0.006	0.084 ±0.005	0.047 ±0.007
Melanoma-skin	1.095 ±0.132	1.051 ±0.137	1.209 ±0.154	0.845 ±0.075	1.010 ±0.154	0.749 ±0.068
Normal-skin	0.401 ±0.055	0.256 ±0.055	0.286 ±0.058	0.090 ±0.009	0.122 ±0.018	0.071 ±0.008
Cornea	0.834 ±0.269	0.173 ±0.102	0.891 ±0.717	0.200 ±0.059	0.084*	0.062
Lens	0.017 ±0.013	0.023 ±0.012	0.021 ±0.017	0.005 ±0.006	0.006*	0.005
Vitreous	0.031 ±0.016	0.028 ±0.007	0.036 ±0.015	0.031 ±0.012	0.014*	0.018
Retina	0.169 ±0.106	0.074 ±0.007	0.251 ±0.132	0.206 ±0.002	0.091*	0.127
Choroid	1.109 ±0.631	0.950 ±0.855	0.337 ±0.163	0.361 ±0.103	0.127*	0.131 ±0.124
Kidney	25.32 ±2.55	18.156 ±1.205	17.703 ±2.069	10.508 ±0.481	17.443 ±1.766	3.904 ±0.217
Liver	5.463 ±0.721	4.273 ±0.350	7.188 ±0.701	3.729 ±0.346	4.841 ±0.398	2.331 ±0.457
Gonads	2.076 ±1.017	0.238 ±0.041	0.663 ±0.142	0.164 ±0.029	0.135 ±0.020	0.079 ±0.004
Brain	0.107 ±0.025	0.067 ±0.006	0.135 ±0.123	0.139 ±0.019	0.067* ±0.008	0.109 ±0.010
Muscle	0.159 ±0.024	0.100 ±0.020	0.090 ±0.015	0.026 ±0.003	0.041 ±0.005	0.027 ±0.011
Blood	3.870 ±0.749	3.635 ±0.404	5.847 ±0.828	3.007 ±0.267	3.792 ±0.224	0.852 ±0.175
Bone	3.977 ±0.648	3.991 ±0.641	5.320 ±0.717	5.342 ±0.758	9.761 ±2.016	5.757 ±0.602
Intestines	0.841 ±0.238	0.653 ±0.111	1.593 ±0.265	1.664 ±0.457	2.064* ±0.597	0.217 ±0.095

[a] Averages and standard deviations for an average of 8–17 hamsters per time group, except data marked*, which represent results from 4 animals.

that melanoma imaging with ^{203}Pb-tris is feasible. Figure 3 is a scan taken with a Nuclear Data gamma camera with a pinhole collimator, at 24 hours after an intraperitoneal injection of 50 μCi of ^{203}Pb-tris. The arrow is pointing to the area of an ocular melanoma.

A more limited analysis of ^{57}Co-bleomycin and thallium-201 chloride is given in Tables 2 and 3. The ratio of ^{57}Co-bleomycin in eye melanoma to choroid of ∼3.8 is favor-

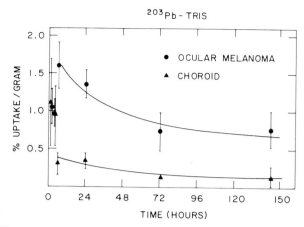

Fig. 2.   Uptake of ^{203}Pb-tris in the ocular melanoma and choroid of the hamster at 1 to 144 hours.

able. The ratio of tumor to choroid was similar to the ^{203}Pb-tris. However, the ratio of percent uptake per gram in the tumor eye to normal eye was significant, that is, $\sim$ 57 to 1. However the percent uptake of the labeled bleomycin (0.52 $\pm$ 0.14 %/g) is not so great as for the ^{203}Pb-tris (1.61 $\pm$ 0.32 %/g) (Fig. 4). The percent uptake of thallium-201 in skin melanoma is lower, and the ratio of uptake in melanoma to skin is unfavorable for detection. There was greater uptake of thallium-201 in the normal eye than with the other labeled compounds tested.

DISCUSSION

The Greene melanoma was selected because of its degree of pigmentation, and initially radiopharmaceuticals with pigment affinity were investigated for melanoma localization, that is, quinoline analogs. Therefore, comment cannot be made as to amelanotic melanoma and the compounds that we have used. In addition, human confirmation is necessary.

Heavy metals have been previously found in higher concentration in neoplastic tissue,[6, 7] although these findings have not been consistent.[10, 11] The studies were performed with different tumor models, that is mammary carcinoma[10] and S-91 melanoma.[7] A factor that may lead to lead-203 localizing in a melanotic tumor is the findings of Browness[9] that metals associate with melanin and a melanin-protein complex. Lead-203 tris has also been found to localize to varying degrees in other tumor models[15] in mice, including ependymoma and adenocarcinoma of the breast.

Potts found that thallous ion concentrated in melanin-containing tissues.[14] Table 3 shows that the concentration of thallium-201 in melanoma is not so great as either ^{203}Pb-tris or ^{57}Co-bleomycin. Potts[14] also found a high lens concentration of thallium, whereas our data show a low lens concentration of ^{203}Pb-tris (Table 1). Thus, it would appear that ^{203}Pb-tris is more appropriate for ocular tumor localization than thallium-201-chloride.

Bleomycin, as a prototype antibiotic with tumor affinity was investigated with the ^{57}Co label because of its availability. Cobalt-57 has a long half-life (271 days) and is not

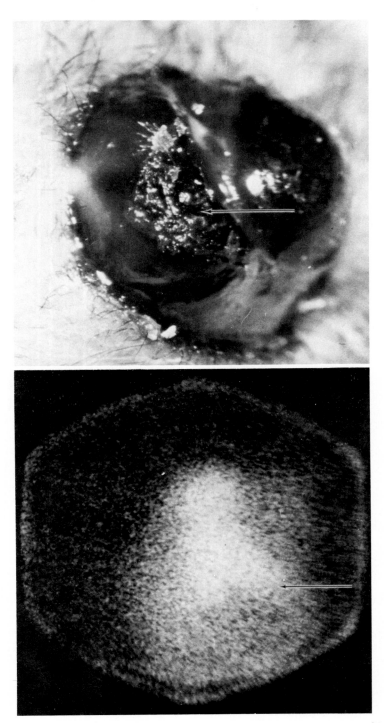

Fig. 3. Scintiphoto and photo of the ocular Greene melanoma in the hamster at 24 hours post intraperitoneal administration. The arrows indicate the location of the tumor.

TABLE 2. DISTRIBUTION OF ^{57}CO-BLEOMYCIN IN PERCENT UPTAKE PER GRAM OF TISSUE AT VARIOUS TIMES[a,b]

Tissue	Time				
	1	3	6	24	144
Melanoma-eye		0.220 ±.217	0.518 ±.141	0.422 ±.049	0.003 ±.003
Normal-eye	0.076 ±.006	0.008 ±.003	0.009 ±.003	0.0024 ±.0004	0.001 ±.000
Melanoma-skin	1.344 ±.218	0.363 ±.185	0.358 ±.30	0.211 ±.067	0.003 ±.002
Normal-skin	1.089 ±.486	0.161 ±.328	0.085 ±.037	0.016 ±.007	0.003 ±.000
Cornea		0.160	0.053	0.007	—[c]
Lens		0.003	0.003	0.002	—[c]
Vitreous		0.011	0.006	0.001	0.001
Retina		0.002	0.004	0.009	0.003
Choroid		0.077	0.135	0.064	0.003
Kidney	1.567 ±.376	0.038 ±.020	0.259 ±.031	0.140 ±.020	0.021 ±.005
Liver	0.431 ±.021	0.088 ±.065	0.188 ±.056	0.101 ±.024	0.009 ±.003
Gonads	0.381 ±.077	0.013 ±.012	0.020 ±.005	0.156 ±.122	0.003 ±.001
Brain		0.005 ±.004	0.004 ±.002	0.003 ±.001	
Muscle	0.101 ±.004	0.189 ±.012	0.013 ±.004	0.002 ±.000	0.001 ±.000
Blood	0.446 ±.088	0.017 ±.008	0.006 ±.001	0.002 ±.001	
Bone	0.044 ±.027	0.006 ±.002	0.017 ±.005	0.007 ±.002	0.006 ±.001
Intestines	0.389 ±.013	0.055 ±.016	0.241 ±.036	0.069 ±.027	0.002 ±.001

[a] Average and standard deviation for 3 to 5 animals per group, data grouped.

[b] Loading dose = 0.1 unit per kg body weight.

[c] Less than 0.000 %/g for parts of the eye. See text.

the most suitable for a widespread clinical use. Table 2 and Fig. 4 show that ^{57}Co-bleomycin and ^{203}Pb-tris both exhibit ocular tumor specificity.

It then appears that there are several compounds which have adequate melanoma specificity to allow detection when combined with the appropriate radionuclide. Each appears to have its own in vivo time course probably due to differences in selective partitioning and/or due to different metabolic breakdown. Imaging is best performed when the difference between tumor concentration versus background concentration is adequate (Fig. 3). All the data obtained serve as a basis for appropriate clinical application.

The problem of detecting ocular melanoma involves not only the tumor specifity of compound but also its detectability, that is, is the energy emitted appropriate for count-

TABLE 3. DISTRIBUTION OF CARRIER-FREE THALLIUM-201 CHLORIDE IN PERCENT UPTAKE PER GRAM OF TISSUE AS A FUNCTION OF TIME[a]

Tissue	Time, hr						
	1	3	6	24	48	72	144
Normal-eye	0.239	0.321	0.479	0.456	0.354	0.295	0.119
	±.037	±.038	.067	±.038	±.100	±.028	±.034
Melanoma-skin	0.327	0.718	0.982	0.478	0.389	0.299	0.128
	±.062	±.269	±.159	±.057	±.132	±.036	±.063
Normal-skin	0.225	0.295	0.283	0.190	0.164	0.143	0.047
	±.121	±.079	±.048	±.039	±.055	±.025	±.011
Kidney	12.177	17.904	17.931	10.732	6.047	4.430	2.301
	±2.136	±2.192	±.378	±4.267	±1.484	±.481	±0.947
Liver	2.736	1.806	1.567	0.798	0.649	0.465	0.196
	±.055	±.090	±.120	±.151	±.135	±.091	±.035
Muscle	2.287	0.354	0.805	0.699	0.409	0.461	0.216
	±.846	±.038	±.142	±.110	±.137	±.111	±.058
Blood	1.004	0.144	0.488	0.069	0.073	0.074	0.030
	±.486	±.048	±.071	±.005	±.036	±.023	±.013
Bone	0.283	0.358	0.507	0.703	0.598	0.499	0.226
	±.075	±.182	±.038	±.083	±.161	±.230	±.070
Intestines	4.309	3.033	2.011	1.387	0.661	0.487	0.219
	±.053	±1.566	±.273	±.506	±.102	±.117	±.034

[a] Four hamsters per group.

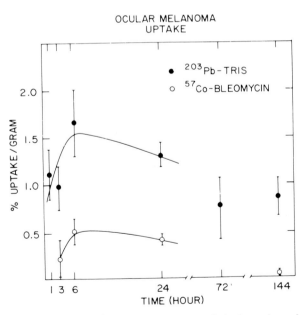

Fig. 4. A comparison of the uptake of [203]Pb-tris and [57]Co-bleomycin in the ocular melanoma as a function of time.

ing or imaging. Very low energy gamma emitters do not have sufficient tissue penetration. Lead-203 [T $\frac{1}{2}$ = 52.1 hours; γ = 279 keV (95%)] or iodine-123 (T $\frac{1}{2}$ = 13.3 hours; γ = 159 keV) should allow for scintigraphy if tumor uptake is adequate. High purity iodine-123 and lead-203 have nuclear decay characteristics appropriate for nuclear ophthalmology. The matrix into which either nuclide is incorporated and its biological behavior will determine which nuclide and compounds are preferable. Since several days must elapse before the ratio of tumor concentration to background is great enough to allow detection, the 13.1 hour half-life of iodine-123 may be less desirable than the 52.1 hour half-life of ^{203}Pb. Lead-203 and ^{123}I have physical half-lives which favor an observation time at 75.2 hours and 18.9 hours, respectively, after administration of the labeled compounds to the patient.

SUMMARY

An experimental procedure has been established to evaluate radiopharmaceuticals for the specific purpose of melanoma detection. By using the Greene melanoma in the hamster, several labeled compounds were compared. Specifically the tumor uptake along with detailed analyses of uptake by various parts of the eye and body were determined in a hamster model. Of those short-lived radionuclides investigated in this laboratory, ^{203}Pb-tris is the most promising as a noninvasive localizing agent for ocular melanoma, and it should allow for ocular scintigraphy.

ACKNOWLEDGMENT

The author gratefully acknowledges the diligent editorial and clerical help of Mrs. Cornelia Osborn.

REFERENCES

1. Hoffer, P. B., and Gottschalk, A.: Tumor Scanning Agents. Sem. Nucl. Med. **4**:305–316 (1974).
2. Wagner, H. N., Jr., and Emmons, H.: In Andrews, G. A., Krisley, R. M., and Wagner, H. N., Jr., Eds., *Radioactive Pharmaceuticals,* U.S. Atomic Energy Commission, Washington, D.C., 1966, pp. 1–32.
3. Lillian, D. L.: The Current Status of Tumor Imaging. *J.A.M.A.* **230**:735–738 (1974).
4. Blanquet, P., and Safi, A.: Diagnosis and Evaluation of Endocular Tumors by Means of Nuclear Indicators. *Int. J. Appl. Rad. Isot.* (in press).
5. Packer, S., Redvanly, C., Wolf, A. P., and Atkins, H. L.: Quinoline Analog Labeled with Iodine-123 in Melanoma Detection. *Arch. Ophthalmol.* (accepted for publication, 1973).
6. Dines, D. E., Elveback, L. R., and McCall, J. T.: Zinc, Copper, and Iron Contents of Pleural Fluid in Benign and Neoplastic Disease. *Mayo Clinic Proc.* **49**:102–106 (1974).
7. O'Rourke, J. F., Patton, H., and Bradley, R.: A Study of the Uptake of ^{32}P, ^{65}Zn and ^{131}I Serum Albumin by Experimental Malignant Melanoma. *Am. J. Ophthalmol.* **44**:190–197 (1957).
8. Packer, S., Lambrecht, R. M., Merrill, J. C., Atkins, H. L., and Wolf, A. P.: Localization of Lead-203 in Ocular and Skin Melanoma (to be published).
9. Browness, J. M., and Morton, R. A.: The Association of Zinc and Other Metals with Melanin and a Melanin-Protein Complex. *Biochem. J.* **53**:620–626 (1953).
10. Caussey, G. The Distribution of Lead After Intravenous Injection in the Tissue of the Rabbit and Tumor-bearing Mice. *Br. J. Cancer* **19**:867 (1965).
11. Beierwaltes, W. H., and Knorpp. C. T. Lack of Selective Uptake of Radioactive Iodine, Phosphorus and Copper by Melanomas in Mouse and Man. *J. Lab. Clin. Med.* **38**:786–787 (1951).

12. Merrill, J. C., Lambrecht, R. M., and Wolf, A. P. Cyclotron Production of Lead-203 for Radiopharma-
     ceutical Applications. *Int. J. Appl. Rad. Isotopes* **24**:701–702 (1973).

13. Greene, H. S. N.: A Spontaneous Melanoma in the Hamster with a Propensity for Amelanotic Altera-
     tion and Sarcomatous Transformation During Transplantation. *Cancer Res.* **18**:422–425 (1958).

14. Potts, A. M., and Au, P. C. Thallous Ion and the Eye. *Invest. Ophthalmol.* **10**:925–931 (1971).

15. Lambrecht, R. M., Bradley-Moore, P. R. et al: Unpublished results. See New Cyclotron Nuclides for
     Radiopharmaceuticals: Titantium-45 and Lead-203. *J. Nucl. Med.* **15**:475–476 (1974).

An Ultrasonic Guided Gamma Probe for Intraocular Melanoma Detection

Michael A. Wainstock, M.D.
Clinical Assistant Professor in Ophthalmology,
Director of Ultrasonic Laboratory,
University of Michigan Medical Center,
Ann Arbor, Michigan

W. Leslie Rogers, Ph.D.
Assistant Professor of Internal Medicine,
Division of Nuclear Medicine,
University of Michigan Medical Center,
Ann Arbor, Michigan

The use of a directional ultrasound probe in combination with a melanoma specific radionuclide such as ^{125}I chloroquine analog is a rational approach to noninvasive techniques for intraocular tumor detection. Beierwaltes and co-workers[1] in 1969 reported on the use of ^{125}I chloroquine analog for the detection of ocular melanoma. With the use of a specially designed handheld probe,[2] it was found possible to detect differential counts between a normal eye and one with suspected melanoma. It was found that concentration of the analog in melanomas increased over normal tissue in a 14-day period with a minimum differentiation of 30%. Unfortunately, amelanotic melanomas (Figs. 1 and 2) showed only a 5–6% differential count in this time period. Inflammatory lesions showed a similar drop-off in count rate differential as has been reported by other authors[3] with radiophosphorus techniques. In the case of chloroquine analog, counting is usually done 4 to 5 days after the oral dose is administered when the general background count has decreased and the concentration in melanomas has increased from 10 to 60 times over that in normal skin, muscle, and fat (Fig. 3 A and B). Rarely does the count rate differential in normal tissue exceed 16%. Table 1 lists a group of pseudomelanomas in which the differential uptake was invariably less then 18%. Those with proven melanomas showed a minimum of 24% differential uptake and averaged 60%.

The use of ultrasound as a diagnostic modality in ophthalmology is well established. The use of "A" and "B" scan modes has been thoroughly outlined by numerous authors. The basic system consists of a handheld transducer probe which is placed against the closed lid with the use of coupling gel and rotated directionally until cross-sectional areas of information through the globe or orbit are obtained. The more sophisticated Jackson-Coleman apparatus (Fig. 4 A and B) requires a water bath immersion of the globe and gives three-dimensional information of better technical quality. Figure 5 is a typical compound scan of a normal eye showing the cornea, lens, vitreous, and retrobulbar fat. In Fig. 6, an unsuspected melanoma hidden by a retinal detachment is easily demonstrated (a is the retinal detachment, b the unsuspected melanoma).

In order to accomplish the task of combining a radionuclide ultrasound probe with a radionuclide detector, it was necessary to miniaturize the components. The radionuclide detector probe is 1 in. in diameter and the collimator consists of 100 hexagonal tubes 1.5 cm long and 0.0015 cm (1 mil) in thickness wrapped with silver foil (Figs. 7 and 8). The line spread function of the collimator is 5 mm FWHM for a standard source 30 mm from the collimator. There are plans to improve this line spread to less than 2 mm,

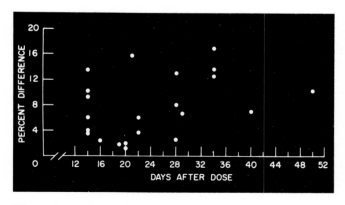

Fig. 1.   Percent difference in counting rate between eyes in control patients.

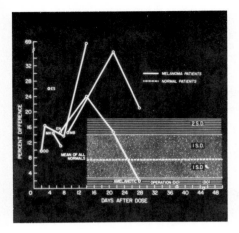

Fig. 2. Mean percent difference in counting rates between the eyes in patients with ocular melanomas and in patients with nonocular melanomas.

TABLE 1. PATIENTS WITH SUSPECTED MELANOMA LESIONS OF THE EYE (GROUP I)

Patient	Clinical or pathological diagnosis	Maximum percent difference after 14 days
Nonmelanoma Lesions		
MP	Kuhnt-Junius degenerative disease	—8%
CB	Metastatic breast carcinoma	3%
SB	Coloboma	15%
JP	Chorioretinitis	10%
FR	Retinal detachment	12%
EA	Retinal vein occlusion	5%
WG	Pigmented nevus	2%
CML	Pigmented nevus	0%
EB	Iris pigmentation (normal variant)	2%
SG	Nonspecific inflammation	17%
LT	Pigmented scar	14.8%
Ocular Melanomas		
MB	Malignant melanoma, OD	48%
EN	Choroidal melanoma, OS	24%
DO	Conjunctival melanoma, OD	69%
OT	Choroidal melanoma, OS	—
MK	Choroidal melanoma, OS	—
ES	Melanoma of ciliary body and peripheral choroid, OD	—

125

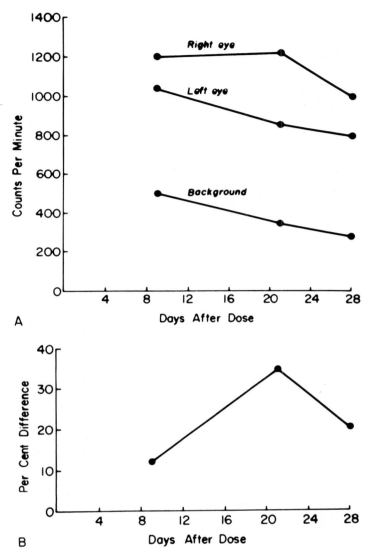

Fig. 3.   *A* shows serial counting rates over eyes in Patient EN studies over 28-day period. *B* shows percent difference in counting rates between eyes of Patient EN over 28-day period.

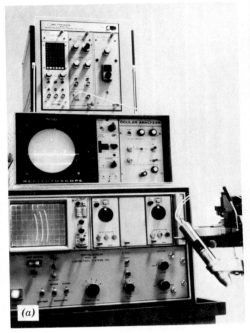

Fig. 4.   (a) Jackson-Coleman Ultrasound Apparatus   (b) Ultrasound waterbath apparatus

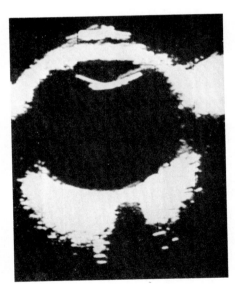

Fig. 5.   Normal ultrasound scan of the globe

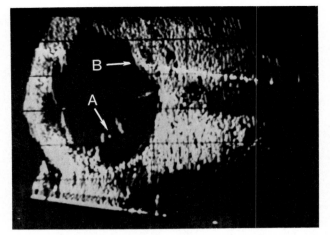

Fig. 6.   Unsuspected melanoma, (A) retinal detachment, (B) melanoma

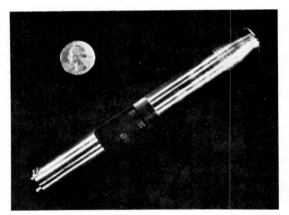

Fig. 7.   Miniaturized radionuclide detection probe.

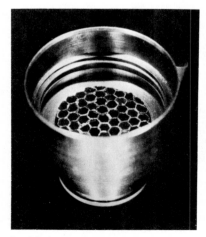

Fig. 8.   Miniaturized radionuclide detection probe.

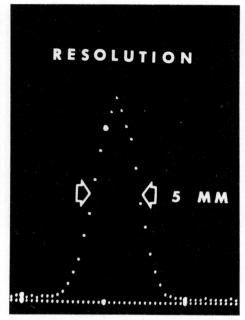

Fig. 9.   Line spread function of collimator.

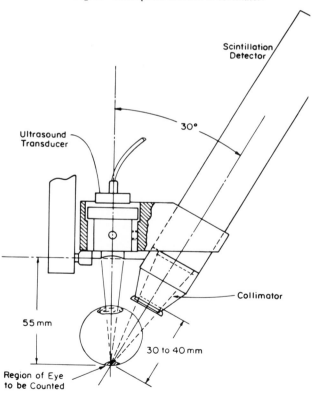

Fig. 10.   Physical characteristics of ultrasonic probe and scintillation detector in combination.

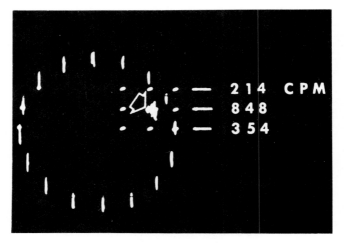

Fig. 11.   Phantom eye.

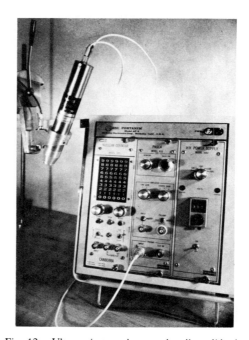

Fig. 12.   Ultrasonic transducer and radionuclide detector probe.

which should be sufficient for accurate localization of smaller tumors (Fig. 9). The ultrasound probe (Fig. 10) has a 10 MHz crystal with a focal length of 55 mm. The focal length of the probe is 30 mm. The focal length may be varied by using crystals of differing energy from 5 MHz to 20 MHz.

Figure 11 demonstrates a "phantom eye" consisting of 16 nylon threads in the form of a tube 2.5 cm in length. A capillary tube containing 0.8 μCi of ^{125}I chloroquine is located at a point inside the tube. The three intensified points in the illustration are produced by a range marker wired into the "M" mode dead switch of the instrument panel which generates three intensified points along the sweep of the ultrasonic beam. The central point indicates the intersection of the probe axis with the sound beam. The other two points are used to identify the general direction of the beam. A marked decrease in counts occurs within 5 mm of the source.

The ultrasound transducer (a) in combination with the radionuclide detector probe (b) are demonstrated in operation in Fig. 12. The hand potentiometer with its crystal may be moved to any new area within 1 or 2 mm of its original position for recounting adjacent or tumor areas.

Although clinical evaluation with the apparatus has not yet been undertaken, it is hoped that shortly the usefulness of this diagnostic tool will be demonstrated and that surgical intervention for melanoma detection with radiophosphorous may no longer always be necessary.

REFERENCES

1. Counsell, R. E. et al: Tumor Localizing Human Malignant Iodinated Quinoline Derivatives. *J. Pharm. Sci.* **56**:1042 (1967).
2. Beierwaltes, W. H., Lieberman, L. M., Varma, V. M. et al: Visualizing Human Malignant Melanoma and Metastases. J.A.M.A. **206**:97–102 (1968).
3. Boyd, C. M. et al: 125-I-Labeled Chloroquin Analog in the Diagnosis of Ocular Melanomas. *J. Nucl. Med.* **12**(9):601–605 (September 1971).

Ocular Scintigraphy

Paul Blanquet, M.D.
Director, de L'Unite de Recherches,
Inserm,
Bordeaux, France

N. Safi, M.D.
Hôpital Pellegrin
Service des Isotopes
Place Amelie Raba-Leon
Bordeaux, France

M. J. LeRebeller, M.D.
Service d'Ophthalmologie,
Hôpital Saint-Andre,
Bordeaux, France

The diagnosis of intraocular tumors presents many difficulties, especially when it requires a surgical procedure. Radionuclidic procedures and echographic techniques have been used as valuable diagnostic aids, especially when enucleation must be considered. Among the radionuclides, the beta emitter ^{32}P has been extensively used since 1953. Although a good tumor marker, radiophosphorus has the drawback of tissue absorption of its beta radiation as well as difficult and unreliable external detection. This was particularly evident in the case of the detection of tumors in the posterior pole of the eye and explains the limited use of the procedure at present. The use of gamma emitters brought a marked improvement in external detection, but required a compound with specific affinity for tumors. . . The detection had to eliminate the gamma radiation taken up by the neighboring tissues (i.e., the anterior cerebral zone). Trevor-Roper and his associates used labeled diiodofluorescein, while Filippone employed serum albumin or fibrinogen labeled with [125]I. Our own experience in this field dates from 1968, when we started to use ^{131}I-diiodofluorescein for eye scanning.

MATERIAL AND METHODS

The practice of radionuclidic scanning of the eye requires an adaptation of the ancillary equipment to the anatomic condition of the eyes.

The Detector

The symmetry of the eyes requires simultaneous detection whether for topographic or quantitative purposes. Our preference has always been for the Anger-type scintillation camera with a crystal of 28 cm diameter.*

Since the labeled diiodofluorescein remains in the eye for a limited period of time, the use of the camera created considerable difficulties in obtaining a reliable image. In order to solve this difficulty, we coupled the camera to an analyzer circuit composed of a double-amplitude coder, a 4096 channel memory block, and a visualization unit.† This system allowed storage of the information as well as quantification and visual display of the stored image.

The Collimator

The collimator is the central element of the detection system. It must be specially adapted to the anatomic condition of the eye. The model we used from the outset had two stenopeic apertures facing each eye; the openings were cylindro-conical in shape with inverse projection; the outer diameter measured 12 mm, while the inner diameter measured 3 mm. The distance between the two openings was fixed at the average interpupillary distance of 75 mm. Furthermore, the collimator had a concave surface adapted to the convexity of the forehead and the nose root of the patient. The thickness of the collimator (170 mm) absorbed any radiation emitted by the juxtaocular regions (cheek, malar region, and temporal zone) (Fig. 1).

However, this first device presented two shortcomings which sometimes resulted in

* PHO GAMMA II and III—Searle Radiographies.
† INTERTECHNIQUE—Plaisir, 78. (France).

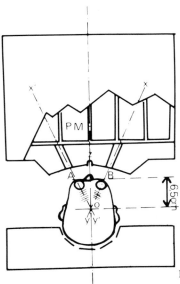

Fig. 1. Collimator No. 1—the distance between the two stenopeic apertures is fixed.

faulty images. The first fault lay in the fixed distance between the two apertures. Thus, when the interpupillary distance differed from the fixed value of 75 mm, the images were no longer centered and the possibility existed that the scanned image could be partially cut off. In addition, the detected areas were not limited to the posterior area of the eye and some cerebral radioactivity was added to the ocular radioactivity. This is represented graphically in Fig. 1 with the shaded areas showing the cerebral regions included in the ocular scan. Fortunately, the cavernous sinuses are located at a considerable distance to the rear of the detected field and do not contribute to the background radiation.

A newly built collimator corrected these disadvantages. The eccentric apertures shown in Fig. 2 made possible the variation of the interpupillary distance between 50 and 80 mm. The shaded areas on the diagram indicate the two mobile parts which may turn freely within their recesses. By rotating each part, it is possible to adapt the apertures to the patient's interpupillary distance.

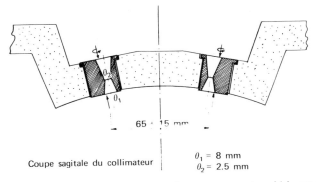

Coupe sagitale du collimateur $\theta_1 = 8$ mm
$\theta_2 = 2.5$ mm

Fig. 2. Collimator No. 2—the shaded areas correspond to tungsten parts, which can turn freely in their lodgement. So the distance between the apertures can be exactly adapted to the interpupillar distance.

The stenopeic apertures have the same conico-cylindrical shape with inverse projection. The outer diameter measures 8 mm and the inner diameter is reduced to 2.5 mm. The axes corresponding to the two stenopeic apertures meet in a focal point situated 35 mm from the tangent plane to the ocular globes (Fig. 3). It is essential to place the collimator in actual contact with the eyes in order to obtain the maximum information.

The reduction of the inner diameter of the apertures to 2.5 mm results in a slight decrease of the efficiency of the system. This can be easily corrected by increasing the amount of ^{131}I-DIF administered to the patient, usually 400 μCi instead of 250–300 μCi. This loss in efficiency is compensated by a significant increase in the resolving power of the system. Indeed, with the former cylindro-conic collimator, the resolution could not exceed the limit of 7–8 mm, even under the best conditions. The present pinhole collimator can resolve 3 mm, and it may surpass this limit. This was demonstrated by placing a phantom composed of nylon threads impregnated with ^{131}I and separated by a distance of 3 mm between each thread. The results, presented in Fig. 4, show a very good resolution of the thread images (Fig. 5).

The other deficiency of the former collimator is also solved with the new pinhole collimator. The background activity originating from the two anterior cerebral lobes is markedly reduced. This was demonstrated by placing a point source of ^{131}I at the tangent plane of the new collimator. A comparison of the isoresponse curves is shown in Figs. 6 and 7. The curves gave a reduction of the initial radioactivity to 12% at a distance of 27 mm, with further decrease to 8% at 32 mm and 6.5% at 35 mm (Fig. 7).

Radiopharmaceuticals Used

The following radiopharmaceuticals were used for this study.

^{131}*I-Diiodofluorescein (DIF).* ^{131}I-DIF is closely related to fluorescein, currently used in ophthalmology for angiography. It is particularly suited for irrigation studies.

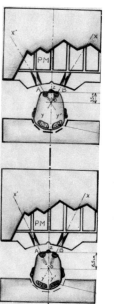

Collimator No. 2
(35 mm)

Collimator No. 1
(65 mm)

Fig. 3.   Comparison between (a) collimator No. 1 (65 mm) and (b) collimator No. 2 (35 mm). The axes corresponding to the two stenopeic apertures meet in a focal point situated 65 mm form the tangent plan to the ocular globes for collimator No. 1 and 35 mm for collimator No. 2.

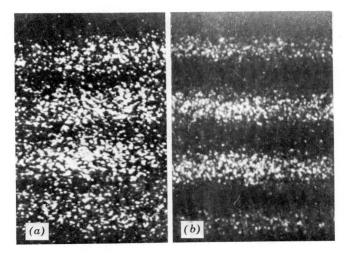

Fig. 4. Compared resolution of collimator No. 1 (*a*) and collimator No. 2 (*b*). The phantom was constituted by nylon threads impregnated with NAI-131 and separated by a distance of 3 mm.

A preliminary study on the kinetics of the eye was carried out with ^{131}I-DIF injected intravenously. The radioisotope uptake was measured with a miniature scintillation detector (NaI), equipped with a conical collimator having an inner diameter of 10 mm and an outer diameter of 3 mm. The highest uptake was noted at 2 to 3 minutes after intravenous injection of the labeled drug. The descendent portion of the radioactivity curve can be divided into three segments indicating respectively:

1. The arteriovenous transit;
2. The invasion of the anterior chamber of the eye;
3. The plateua indicating the equilibrium between plasma and eye activity, continuing at the same level for the remaining period of observation.

Technetium 99m—Pertechnetate. This radiopharmaceutical has been used only recently, together with a collimator of pure tungsten of a diameter of 2.5 mm, specially adapted to the 140 keV radiation of ^{99m}Tc.

Labeled pertechnetate is an excellent indicator of organ perfusion and has the same ocular clearance as that of ^{131}I-DIF. Moreover, the short physical half-life of ^{99m}Tc

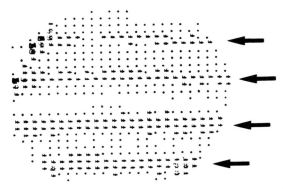

Fig. 5. Resolution of collimator No. 2 "seen" in a computer (3 mm between the arrows).

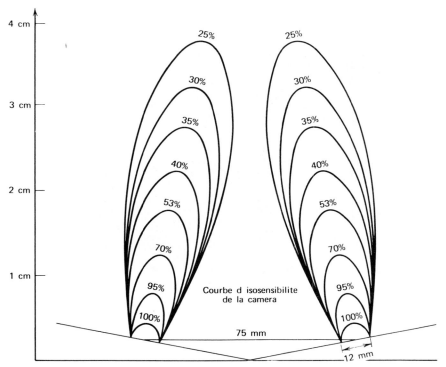

Fig. 6.   Collimator No. 1.

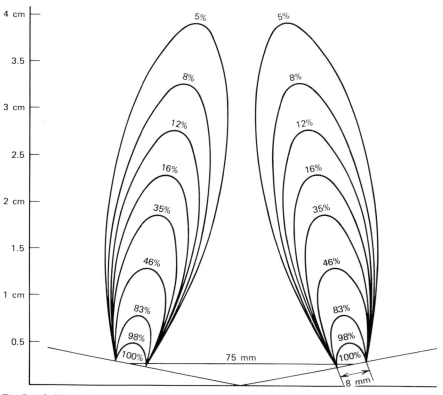

Fig. 7.   Collimator No. 2.

138

allows the administration of higher doses, thus resulting in better statistical results and quantification of the obtained data.

[131]I-iodinated Chloroquine and Chlorpromazine.

The iodinated chloroquine was prepared in our laboratory at approximately the same time as that of Beierwaltes and his associates. The present procedure used in our laboratory is carried out with chloramine-T according to the technique used by Hunter and Greenwood.* A purification of the solution through a column of anionic resin is followed by sterilization through a filtering membrane. The iodination yield rate averages 60% before purification; after purification, free iodine did not exceed 5% of the total radiopharmaceutical. In our experimental conditions, the average specific activities range from 30–40 μCi/mg.

The labeled compound must be used within a short time after preparation, since it undergoes rapid decomposition with release of free iodine. After 3 days of preservation at + 4°C, the amount of free iodine may reach 25%. After administration to the hamster, it was noted that the compound was selectively concentrated in the melanotic tumors, that is, in the induced solid tumors of the Moore strain. The maximum uptake was noted in the third to the fourth days after administration. The administration of labeled ^{131}I-iodochloroquine was first carried out by Blois and his associates and by Beierwaltes and his colleagues. Our own experience in humans started shortly afterwards.

Scanning Technique

Before the administration of iodinated compounds, the thyroid of the patient is blocked with Lugol's solution administered three days preceding the test.

The patient is placed in the supine position, and the ocular globes are in contact with the collimator. For accurate positioning, the image of a luminous guide (Z in Fig. 1), located on the symmetrical axis of the collimator, must form clearly at the nose-root level. The ocular globes must remain immobile throughout the examination, in order to avoid blurring of the image.

After intravenous injection of ^{131}I-DIF or of ^{99m}Tc-pertechnetate, information is stored for 25 to 30 minutes in the 4096 channel-memory and visualized on the screen; images can be obtained with Polaroid photos.

A scintigraphic image of a normal eye is shown in Fig. 8, following intravenous administration of [99m]Tc. The ocular images consist of bright dots and show two oval-shaped areas, indicating an almost equal amount of radioactive compound in each eye. Another normal image (^{99m}Tc) is shown in Fig. 9; the picture is slightly defocused, affording a better interpretation than the dotted image.

When an increased vascularization of the eye is suspected, a better display of the image can be obtained by varying the brightness and the contrast of the scan. The threshold of visualization is changed in Fig. 10, obtained after administration of ^{131}I-DIF; it is easy to notice that the vascular perfusion of the right eye is markedly increased.

The data can be easily quantified by demarcation of the ocular area on the circuit's matrix. The total activity of each area is then integrated with the aid of a magnetic tape calculator. A simple formula has been applied by comparing the respective radionuclidic uptake in each eye. If (A) is the uptake in the pathological eye and (A') the uptake in

---

* Patent pending in France: PV 70.11.83.

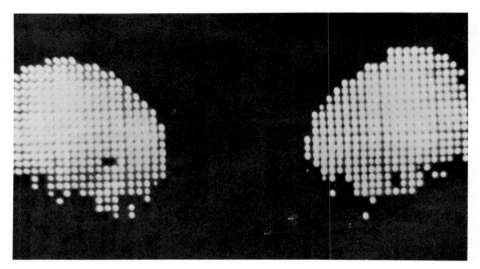

Fig. 8. Normal scintigraphy—(TcO$_4^-$)—NB (the two tiny holes, one on each side are "artifacts" due to the saturation of the memory).

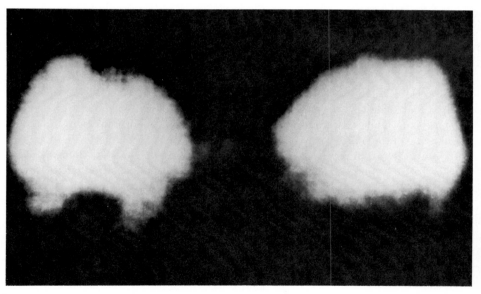

Fig. 9. Normal scintigraphy (TcO^{4-})—the original image has been slightly defocalized. The two ocular areas show essentially the same activity.

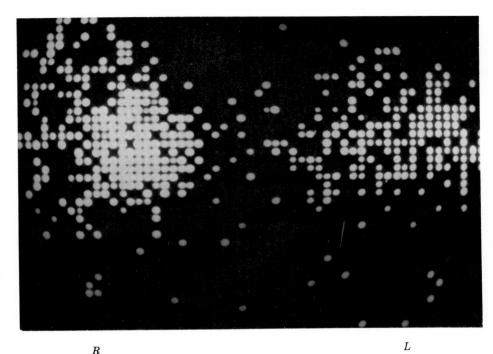

R   L

Fig. 10. Scintigraphy (DIF)—showing an hypervascularization in the right eye. The threshold of the visualization unit has been varied and the dissymmetry appears clearly.

the healthy eye, the ratio between the two eyes can be expressed as

$$K = \frac{(A) - (A')}{(A)} \times 100$$

When scanning is performed with ^{131}I-chloroquine, the examination is made 2 to 3 days after an oral administration of 500 μCi of the labeled compound. Since the iodinated chloroquine is not taken up by the healthy eye, the image obtained is usually unilateral, as shown in Figs. 11 and 12.

RESULTS

Our experience in ocular scanning covers a relatively large group of patients, approximately 500 since 1965. A first group of 198 patients was investigated only with ^{131}I-DIF and had only limited clinical information. In 32 subjects considered normal, the value of the K index ranged between 0 and 14%. In 126 patients with a possibility of a melanotic tumor, the value of K ranged between 21 and 75%; the ratio averaged 16 to 55% in 50 subjects with other types of eye tumors.

These data confirm the general rule that every tumor is accompanied by an increased regional vascularization. However, this is not a specific sign, and the investigation must be completed with other procedures more specific for melanoma. The patients having a K index greater than 15% were subjected to a dual scintigraphy with ^{131}I-DIF and ^{131}I-chloroquine. A second series of 90 patients was examined with both procedures and was

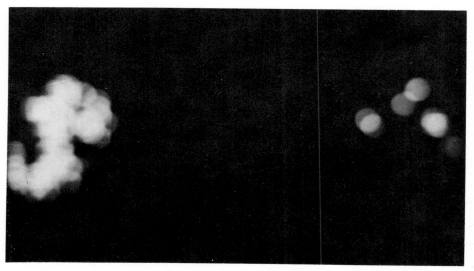

Fig. 11.   Scintigraphy (^{131}I-iodinated chloroquine), showing an important melanotic tumor of the right eye. There is no fixation of the labeled molecule at the level of the left eye.

completed with an extensive clinical study as well as anatomopathological control whenever possible. The results, presented in Table 1, suggest the following comments.

Malignant Melanotic Tumors

The image obtained with ^{131}I-DIF or with ^{99m}TcO$_4^-$ scanning often shows a higher uptake in the region corresponding to the tumor (Fig. 7). Also, the value of K has diagnostic importance as stressed before. In 28 cases of anatomically verified malignant melanomas, K was always above 10% with extreme values ranging between 12 and

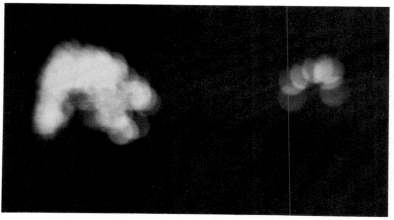

Fig. 12.   Scintigraphy (^{131}I-iodinated chloroquine) showing an important melanotic tumor (crescent-like) of the right eye. As previously, there is no fixation at the level of the left eye.

TABLE 1.   RESULTS: SCINTIGRAPHICAL—CLINICAL—
            ANATOMOPATHOLOGICAL

Number	Classifications	Hypervascularization[a] DIF – ^{99m}Tc	Iodinated Chloroquine	Clinical results	Path. Anat.
5	Angiomas	+ + + +	–	+	
35	Malignant Melanomas	+ + + +	+	+	+
5	Retinoblastomas	+ +	–	+	+
20	Idiopathic Decollements	–	–	+	
20	Choroidites, Benign melanomas	+	–	+	
8	Metastases	+ –	–	+	+

[a] The hypervascularization is indicated as follows: Very important: + + + +: $20\% < K < 65\%$; Medium: + + = $15\% < K < 28\%$; Weak: +: $10\% < K < 20\%$; –: $K < 0$. The negative sign indicates that the activity at the level of the normal eye is more important than at the level of the pathological eye.

75%. The malignant melanoma of the iris always showed a K above 50%, since these tumors are accompanied by early and extensive vascularization.

In 16 cases, scanning with ^{131}I-chloroquine gave a positive image confirmed by anatomopathological data. This is suggestive of a specific uptake of the ^{131}I-chloroquine by the melanotic tumor and also supports the findings of Beierwaltes who noted similar results after external counting procedures with ^{125}I-7-iodoquinoleine. It is hoped that a larger series of cases will confirm these findings and will offer the clinician a test which does not require enucleation.

Benign Melanomas and Choroiditis

Both conditions are accompanied by hyperactive images with a K exceeding 10%, but in these cases there does not seem to be any uptake of ^{131}I-chloroquine. This supports the hypothesis that an uptake of iodinated chloroquine is linked with a sign of malignancy of the melanoma.

Other Tumors or Metastatic Disseminations in the Eye

In this category, the ^{131}I-DIF scanning gives variables results. In sarcomas, the K value is negative, and the scanning shows a low activity with gaps or with unilateral notches. In the four retinoblastomas mentioned in Table 1, the value of K is relatively low, between 15 and 20%; however, the scan suggests a hyperactive area. With metastases of primary tumors, the image may be hyper- or hypoactive. Figure 13 shows the scanning of a bilateral metastasis of a breast cancer, with a markedly active image in the left eye and a relatively less active and lacunar image in the right eye. It must be stressed that the uptake of ^{131}I-chloroquine was negative in each of the metastases and in the other types of neoplasm.

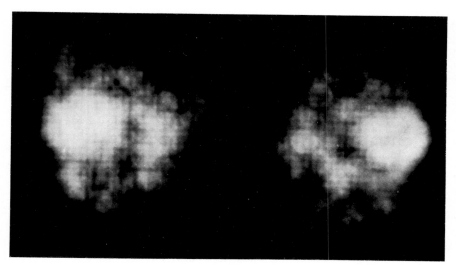

Fig. 13.   Scintigraphy (DIF) showing bilateral metastasis of cancer of the breast.

Idiopathic Retina Detachment

When the detachment is recent, the ^{131}I-DIF scanning shows a loss of activity in the detached portion. This was consistently found in 18 cases. As expected, the ^{131}I-chloroquine uptake was negative. It is important to note that a retina detachment linked with an underlying eye tumor raises serious diagnostic problems.

Other Eye Diseases

In cases of vascular lesions, such as diabetic arteritis or atherosclerosis, the images obtained with ^{131}I-DIF scanning may range from regular and homogeneous scintigrams to bilaterally heterogeneous images. Often, the outlines are blurred and there are many lacunas in the scan.

The images obtained in glaucomas are hyperactive and perfectly homogeneous with sharply delimited outlines and a high K ratio. It seems that the homogeneous scan obtained in a glaucomatous eye has diagnostic importance.

Images obtained in cataracts, pseudotumoral chorioretinitis, and other conditions were negative, both with ^{131}I-DIF as well as with ^{131}I-chloroquine.

DISCUSSION

Equipment

The camera coupled to an analyzer circuit is indispensable, especially when a rapid transit phenomenon is analyzed, such as the blood flow after intravenous injection of ^{131}I-DIF or ^{99m}TcO$_4^-$. Storage of information is also necessary. The analyzer circuit with its matrix permits attainment of accurate data, especially in the integration of the counts and calculation of the K factor.

The resolution of the Anger camera has been improved by the interposition of a light amplifier between the crystal and the phototube. Thus, a resolution of 4 mm can be obtained with a cylindrical collimator; it is possible that the adaptation of the pinhole collimator to the new camera could lower the resolving power to 1.5–2.0 mm.

For static images, (as with ^{131}I-chloroquine) the conventional rectilinear scanning is recommended. At present, we are testing a device composed of two symmetrical detectors with a semimicrocrystal connected by a small light guide to the window of a photomultiplier.

The availability of solid-state detector gave a new impetus to radionuclidic procedures in ophthalmology. In 1971, Larose reported the result of ^{32}P uptake by the eye in different conditions in 122 patients. The measurements were performed with a miniature Geiger probe as well as with different types of solid-state detectors sensitive to beta radiation. The chief disadvantage of both Geiger and solid-state detectors is the marked tissular absorption of beta radiation, necessitating the administration of large amounts of ^{32}P to the patient if a significant uptake is desired in the eye. The patient receives either 10 μCi/kg body weight or a maximum of 700 μCi of a ^{32}PO$_4$ solution by intravenous route and the uptake is measured 48 hours after injection. The dose delivered to the total body is about 1 rad in the first day after injection and about 30 rads to the skeleton. What is even more limiting than the radiation danger is the elaborate and delicate surgical technique required for the placement of the detectors in the optimum position. Nevertheless, in Larose's opinion, the semiconductor offers advantages over the Geiger probe, chiefly because it is possible to obtain a good distinction between signals and background noise, by intercalating an adequate pulse-height analyzer. This feature cannot be obtained with Geiger probes and holds promise for the use of semiconductor probes.

It is doubtful whether the solid-state detectors would become clinically useful if applied only for the beta radiations. As long as an adequate gamma-sensitive solid-state detector is not available, the procedure will remain only an academic speculation. The recent development of gamma-sensitive cadmium-tellurium solid-state detectors constitute a significant advance in this field. Meyer and his associates obtained good results with a CdTe subminiature detector, with a resolution below 2 mm and a maximum signal/noise ratio of 30 or more for gamma energies below 80 keV. While the CdTe probe is less sensitive for the gamma spectrum of ^{131}I, it is perfectly suited to the weak radiation of ^{125}I, as well as to the 140 keV of ^{99m}Tc.

Our present investigation explores the possibility of coupling the CdTe semiconductor to the scintillation camera in order to obtain a better resolution of the image. It must be noted that the CdTe detector requires only a very thin collimator, which makes it more versatile than the pinhole collimator described in this paper.

Collimation

The adjustable collimator adapted to the interpupillary distance of each patient gives satisfactory results. In cases of scanning with ^{99m}Tc, the inner opening could be reduced to 2 mm, resulting in an appreciable improvement in the resolution. Unfortunately, when a scanning with ^{131}I-chloroquine is contemplated the amount of radiopharmaceutical must be substantially increased in order to obtain a good image. This is not desirable, since the amount of labeled compound to be injected is already high. An alternate solution would be to perform the ^{99m}Tc scanning with the 2 mm pinhole collimator and to repeat the scanning with ^{131}I-chloroquine with a larger aperture (2.5–3.0 mm). Obviously, the resolving power will not be identical for each scanning.

Radiopharmaceuticals

The use of ^{131}I-DIF raises few questions, since the diagnostic application of fluorescein is well known by ophthalmologists. Also, the use of ^{99m}TcO$_4^-$ for circulation studies is frequently applied in nuclear medicine.

Conversely, we know little about tumor uptake of iodinated chloroquine or related substances. In fact, we do not know whether the localization is selective for the intact molecule or for a metabolic product of iodinated chloroquine. However, the following few points are known:

1.   The localization of ^{131}I-chloroquine does not appear to be directly linked to the presence of melanin, since achromic melanomas have the same range of uptake as the pigmented melanomas.

2.   The specific localization suggests the action of a complex enzymic system, involving beta glycuronidase, hemopexin, and tyrosinase in particular.

At present, the mechanism of uptake is being studied with chloroquine labeled with ^{131}I and ^{14}C in tissue cultures of human melanomas. It must be added that gallium-67 and bleomycin labeled with ^{57}Co did not give conclusive results. Even in a positive result, the hard gamma radiation of cobalt precludes its utilization for routine diagnosis.

Value and Applications of Eye Scanning

The value of the K coefficient in the diagnosis of ocular pathology appears to be significant, especially in cases where there is an increase of 20% or more. This has been confirmed by numerous clinical and anatomical data. However, there are instances where a high K value is not associated with eye malignancy; there have also been cases with proven malignancies having a K value between 12 and 20% (three cases in our last series). One patient with a hypervascularization associated with a granuloma exhibited a K value higher than 20%. As a rule, we considered as probable malignancy those cases with a K value exceeding 20%, and as suspicious those cases with a lower value of K (15–20%). In these patients, iodochloroquine may offer additional information.

In our experience, eye scanning is a valuable diagnostic tool for the ophthalmologist. It can be applied in the following circumstances.

1.   In cases of visible tumors in the anterior segment of the eye (such as in tumors of the iris, the choroid, or the ciliary body). The clinical diagnosis may already be made, but scanning can give an indication of the degree of vascularization of the tumor; the elevated value of K can alter and can suggest alternate administration of ^{131}I-DIF or ^{99m}TcO$_4^-$. Eye scanning is particularly useful both before and after iridectomy in cases of tumors of the iris.

2.   With tumors situated in the posterior segment, K is high as stated before; furthermore, ^{131}I-chloroquine offers additional information.

3.   When a tumor is suspected, the dual uptake may be of value, especially when the ^{131}I-chloroquine uptake is positive and K has an elevated value; this was highly

suggestive of malignant melanoma in our experience. In high K and a negative
[131]I-chloroquine uptake, there is a possibility of other tumors, such as sarcoma, glioma
of the retina, hemangioma of the choroid, or metastases of other tumors.

Since malignant melanoma may start with a varied symptomatology such as retinal
detachment, intraocular hemorrhage, unilateral glaucoma, or choroiditis, it is suggested
that a dual scintigraphy be performed on patients with this symptomatology, in order to
ascertain the nature of these symptoms.

In conclusion, radionuclidic examination of the eye opens new diagnostic possibilities.
The assessment of eye vascularization and the presence of a tumor with a specific affinity to a labeled compound constitute some of the immediate applications. It is hoped
that with the development of detector technology and especially the understanding of the
biochemical substrate of the uptake of some compounds by the eye malignancies new applications for the diagnosis of eye conditions will result.

ACKNOWLEDGMENT

The help of Mr. Kulberg from Searle Radiographics is gratefully acknowledged.

REFERENCES

1. Appelmans, M., and Wouters, K.: Détection des Tumeurs Malignes de l'Orbite par le Phosphore Radioactif. Congrès Int. Ophtal. (Bruxelles 8–12 Septembre 1958); *C. R. Acta. Conc. Ophtal.* **1**:513–517
   (1959).

2. Bessiere, E., Verin Ph., Le Rebeller, M. J., Descamp, F., Safi, N., and Desme, D.: A Propos de la Scintigraphie Oculaire. *Bull. Ophtal. France* **58**:879–884 (1968).

3. Bettman, J. W.: Radioactive Phosphorus as a Diagnosis Aid in Ophthalmology. *Arch. Ophthalmol.*
   (*Chicago*) **51/2**:172–179 (1954).

4. Blanquet, P., Beck, C., Ducassou, D., Basse-Cathalinat, B., Safi, N., and Vilayleck, S.: Utilisation
   d'une Chaîne d'Analyse Multiparamétrique en Pratique Hospitalière Courante. *I.A.E.A. SM* 136/
   94:125–132 (1971).

5. Blanquet, P., Bessiere, E., Desme, D., Verin, Ph., Le Rebeller, M. J., and Safi, N.: A Propos de la
   Scintigraphie Oculaire. *Bordeaux-Médical* **12**(2):301–308 (1968).

6. Blois, M. S.: Melanin Binding Properties of Iodine. *J. Invest. Dermatol.* **50**:250–253 (1958).

7. Blois, M. S.: The Uptake of Radioactivity Labeled Compounds by Malignant Melanoma. Paper given
   at the XIII Internat. Congress of Dermatol. Munich, July 31–August 5, 1967.

8. Blois, M. S.: Melanoma Detection with Radioiodoquine. *J. Nucl. Med.* **9**:492 (1968).

9. Boyd, C. M., Beierwaltes, W. H., Lieberman L. M., and Bergström, T. J.: [125]I Labeled Chloroquine
   Analog in the Diagnosis of Ocular Melanomas. *J. Nucl. Med.* **12**:601 (1971).

10. Counsell, R. E., Pocha, P., Morales, J. O. and Beierwaltes, W. H.: Tumor Localizing Human Ma-
    lignant Iodinated Quinoline Derivates. *J. Pharm. Sci.* **56**:1042 (1967).

11. Dunphy, E. B.: The Status of Radioactive Phosphorus in the Detection of Ocular Tumor. *Acta XVIII°
    Cong. Ophthalmol.* (1958).

12. Ferny, A. P.: Lesions Mistaken for Malignant Melanoma of the Posterior Uvea: A Clinicopathologic
    Analysis of 100 Cases with Ophthalmoscopically Visible Lesions. *Arch. Ophthalmol.* (*Chicago*) **72**:463
    (1964).

13. Safi, N., Blanquet, P., Verin, Ph., and Moretti, J. L.: Utilisation d'un Nouveau Traceur Radioactif
    dans la Détection des Tumeurs Mélaniques Endoculaires. *Bull. Soc. Ophtal. Franç. Lyon.* (Novembre
    1969).

14. Safi, N.: Utilisation des Indicateurs Nucléaires pour la Détection des Tumeurs Endoculaires. *Thèse de
    Doctorat en Médecine, Bordeaux, 1969.*

15. Safi, N., Blanquet, P., Moretti, J. L., and Verin, Ph.: Utilisation d'un Nouveau Vecteur dans le Diag-
     nostic des Mélanomes. *A.T.E.N.*, **22**:17–20 (1969).

16. Safi, N., Moretti, J. L., Vilayleck, S., and Blanquet, P.: ^{131}I-Iodoquine for Diagnosis and Localization
     of Malignant Melanoma. *J. Nucl. Med.* (September 1970).

17. Safi, N., Blanquet, P., and Rouge, F.: Apport des Molécules Marquées au Diagnostic et à la Sur-
     veillance des Tumeurs Mélaniques. *Biomedicine* **19**:122–125 (1973).

18. Safi, N.: Apport des Molécules Marquées dans l'Étude des Tumeurs Mélaniques Expérimentales et Hu-
     maines. Doctorat d'Etat en Biologie humaine présente et soutenue publiquement à Bordeaux, December
     5, 1974.

Metastatic Disease

Metastatic Tumors to and from the Eye: Clinical and Pathologic Considerations

Jerry A. Shields, M.D.
Senior Assistant Surgeon,
Retina Service,
Wills Eye Hospital,
Philadelphia, Pennsylvania

In a routine practice of ophthalmology, metastatic tumors to and from the eye are rather uncommon. When such a tumor does occur, however, the clinician may be confronted with a number of diagnostic problems and difficult therapeutic decisions. This section considers some important *clinical* and *pathologic* highlights of both metastatic tumors to the eye from distant primary sites and metastatic tumors from the eye to distant organs. Metastatic tumors to and from the orbit and ocular adnexa are not considered here.

METASTATIC TUMORS TO THE EYE

Tumors metastatic to the intraocular structures involve primarily the uveal tract. The choroid is the most common site for metastasis and the anterior uvea is somewhat less commonly involved. Isolated metastasis to the optic nerve and retina are extremely rare. Metastasis to the cornea, sclera, lens, and vitreous probably do not occur.

The tendency for metastasis to involve the choroid may be partially explained by the great vascularity of this tissue. Tumor emboli pass through the internal carotid artery to the ophthalmic artery and finally into the ciliary vessels to settle in the choroid. Despite the general belief that there is a preference for the left eye, recent evidence indicates an equal incidence of metastasis to the right and left eyes.[1]

One of the difficult diagnostic problems that may confront the ophthalmologist is in differentiating a tumor metastatic to the choroid from a primary choroidal melanoma.[2] In many cases, if a metastatic ocular tumor is suspected, a thorough medical evaluation will detect the primary lesion. In some instances, however, the primary site may remain occult.

Although frequent exceptions occur, there are certain ophthalmoscopic features that are useful in making the differentiation between metastatic tumors to the eye and primary choroidal melanomas. Metastatic tumors are usually nonpigmented, or amelanotic, having a white or yellow appearance, often with typical brown pigment clumps on the surface (Fig. 1). A notable exception is the metastatic melanoma to the choroid from skin, which is often pigmented. Primary melanomas usually have some degree of internal pigment and appear black, grey, or mottled brown, with yellow or orange pigment on the surface.[3] Metastatic tumors may sometimes be bilateral, multifocal, multilobed, or diffuse (Fig. 2). The primary melanoma usually occurs as a unilateral isolated lesion. The extent of the associated serous retinal detachment is usually greater with a metastatic tumor than with a primary melanoma. This can be best appreciated with indirect ophthalmoscopy.

In addition to ophthalmoscopy, certain ancillary tests such as ultrasonography[4] and fluorescein angiography[5] may be useful in differentiating these lesions. The radioactive phosphorus (^{32}P) uptake test, although useful in differentiating benign from malignant lesions, is not helpful in differentiating a primary choroidal melanoma from a tumor metastatic to the choroid.[6-11]

The majority of metastatic tumors to the eye are carcinomas. Ferry and Font[1] recently tabulated the incidence of the primary sites for carcinomas metastatic to the intraocular structures (Table 1). The breast is the most common primary site in females and the lung in males. In a substantial number of cases, the primary site is never determined,

From the Oncology Unit, Retina Service, Wills Eye Hospital, Philadelphia, Pennsylvania. Supported in part by the Retina Research and Development Foundation, Philadelphia, and the Lions Club of Pennsylvania.

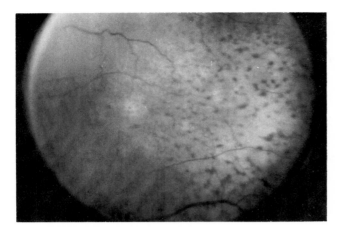

Fig. 1.   Fundus photograph of metastatic tumor to choroid from breast. Note the dark pigment clumping on light background.

either because autopsy was not performed or because medical evaluation failed to locate the "occult" primary lesion. Even a histologic study of the ocular tumor may often fail to define the primary site.

In cases of metastatic breast tumors to the eye, the patient usually has a history of previous mastectomy or a breast mass is found concurrently with the ocular lesion. In cases of metastatic tumors from lung, kidney, or gastrointestinal tract, however, the ocular metastases may sometimes be the initial manifestation of malignancy, and the primary lesion may not become apparent for weeks or months after the ocular symptoms. It has been recently demonstrated that carcinoembryonic antigen (CEA) may be useful in differentiating a metastatic tumor from a primary choroidal melanoma in those cases where a primary malignancy cannot be found.[12, 13]

Other lesions besides amelanotic melanomas may clinically resemble metastatic tu-

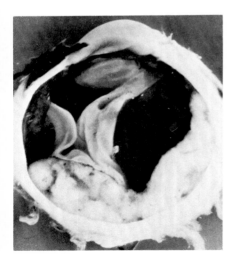

Fig. 2.   Sectioned globe containing metastatic tumor from breast. Note the amelanotic, multinodular tumor with extensive overlying retinal detachment.

TABLE 1.   FOCUS OF PRIMARY TUMOR IN 227
           PATIENTS WITH CARCINOMAS
           METASTATIC TO THE EYE
           (EXPRESSED IN PERCENTAGES)[a, b]

Site of Primary Tumor	Male	Female
Breast	—	78.6
Lung	53.8	11.6
Kidney	7.5	—
Testicle	6.5	—
Prostate	2.2	—
Pancreas	1.1	—
Colon	1.1	1.0
Rectum	1.1	1.0
Stomach	1.1	—
Thyroid	1.1	—
Not determined	24.7	7.8
Total	100	100

[a] Percentages may not add to 100.0 because of rounding.
[b] Modified from reference 1.

mors to the choroid. Various types of choroiditis and episcleritis may produce a yellow choroidal mass and an overlying retinal detachment, resembling a metastatic tumor. Leukemias,[5] lymphomas, and lymphoid hyperplasia[14] may produce a similar ophthalmoscopic picture. When confronted with an amelanotic choroidal mass, the clinician must consider the possibility of a metastatic tumor to the choroid and the clinical evaluation directed accordingly. By proper utilization of modern diagnostic approaches,[15, 16] the ophthalmologist may make the correct diagnosis and refer the patient for chemotherapy or radiation as indicated.

METASTATIC TUMORS FROM THE EYE

Primary intraocular malignant tumors may metastasize to other parts of the body. The malignant melanoma of the uvea and the retinoblastoma are the only two lesions that are common enough to warrant consideration.

Malignant Melanoma

The malignant melanoma of the uvea is the most common primary intraocular malignancy. Malignant melanomas arising from the iris are usually discovered while the tumor is still small and localized. In most cases, they may be excised by a sector iridectomy or iridocyclectomy and the prognosis is usually very good. Those arising from the posterior uvea, however, are usually larger when discovered and have a greater tendency to metastasize. When the patient with a posterior uveal melanoma initially presents to the ophthalmologist, systemic evaluation usually reveals no evidence of

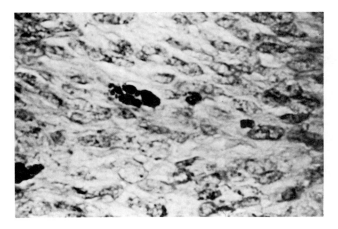

Fig. 3.   Choroidal melanoma with predominantly spindle-cells. (hematoxylin-eosin, × 320).

metastasis. About one-half of patients enucleated for these tumors, however, will eventually develop metastases.[18, 19]

There are several pathologic features that appear related to whether or not an intraocular melanoma will metastasize. These include the cell type, tumor size, degree of extraocular extension, and growth pattern of the tumor.[18] These features may overlap; for example, the tumors with more malignant cell types are more likely to be larger and exhibit extrascleral extension. Other factors, such as degree of pigmentation and reticulin fiber count, are rarely used any longer to predict prognosis. Recent studies have demonstrated tumor-specific antibodies in the plasma of patients with uveal melanomas.[20] One may speculate that a decrease in the level of these circulating antibodies may eventually prove to be related to metastatic disease.

With regard to cell type, uveal melanomas are classified according to the Callender classification.[18] The spindle-cell tumors (Fig. 3) are less likely to metastasize, whereas those tumors containing epithelioid cells (Fig. 4) are more likely to spread. There are

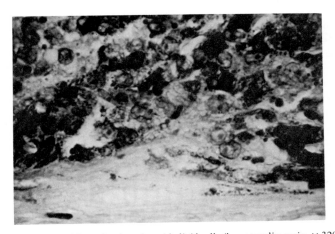

Fig. 4.   Choroidal melanoma with predominantly epithelioid cells (hematoxylin-eosin, × 320).

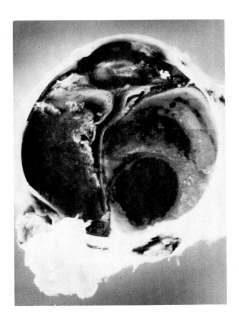

Fig. 5. Sectioned globe filled with large necrotic, hemorrhagic malignant melanoma arising from choroid. Patient developed clinical evidence of metastasis within 1 year after enucleation.

TABLE 2. SITES OF METASTATIC FOCI FROM MALIGNANT MELANOMAS OF THE POSTERIOR UVEA (38 CASES)[a]

Focus	Number	Percent
Liver alone	13	34
Liver plus other organs	24	63
Other organs minus liver	1	3
	38	100
Other Organs		
Pleura plus lungs	13	
Pericardium plus myocardium	9	
Gastrointestinal tract	9	
Lymph nodes	8	
Pancreas	6	
Skin	6	
Central nervous system	4	
Bones	3	
Suprarenal glands	3	
Thyroid gland	2	
Kidneys	2	
Ovaries	2	
Others	3	

[a] Modified from reference 25.

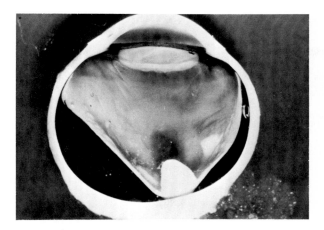

Fig. 6.   Gross speciman of globe showing two small retinoblastomas in posterior pole, not involving optic nerve.

definite exceptions to this generality, however, and even the relatively benign spindle A melanomas have been known to metastasize.[21]

With regard to tumor size, there is good evidence that, in eyes enucleated for posterior uveal melanomas, the incidence of metastases is greater for large tumors than for small tumors (Fig. 5).[21, 22] There is also good evidence that the prognosis is poor in cases with significant extrascleral extension of the tumor.[23] Finally, those tumors that exhibit a diffuse, rather than a focal, growth pattern have a higher incidence of metastasis.[24]

Primary intraocular melanomas may spread either by direct extension to adjacent structures or by hematogenous routes to distant organs. The sites of distant metastasis are shown in Table 2.[25] The liver is the most common metastatic focus, being involved in 97% of all choroidal melanomas that metastasize. Metastasis may also occur to lung, pleura, pericardium, myocardium, gastrointestinal tract, and numerous other sites. Since the liver is involved in 97% of metastatic disease, patients with a history of choroidal melanoma should definitely have periodic liver function studies as part of their medical follow-up evaluation.

Retinoblastoma

The retinoblastoma is the most common primary intraocular tumor in childhood. Its clinical and histologic features are well known.[18, 19] If such a tumor is diagnosed while it is still small, it may be treated with enucleation or radiation and the prognosis is quite favorable (Fig. 6).[26] In those patients who succumb to retinoblastoma, death results from intracranial extension in 50%, from generalized metastasis in 40%, and from extension into the nose and mouth in 10%.[19] Reese has pointed out the foci of metastases from retinoblastoma (Table 3).[19] Skull, long bones, spinal cord, lymph nodes, and viscera are the most common sites.

There are several histopathologic features that are useful as prognostic indicators in retinoblastoma. These include the degree of invasion of the optic nerve, the degree of cellular differentiation, and the presence or absence of choroidal invasion.

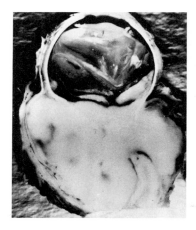

Fig. 7. Gross globe showing retinoblastoma in posterior segment with extensive invasion of orbit and optic nerve.

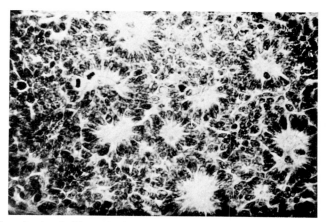

Fig. 8. Well-differentiated retinoblastoma, showing numerous Flexner-Wintersteiner rosettes (hematoxylin-eosin, × 320).

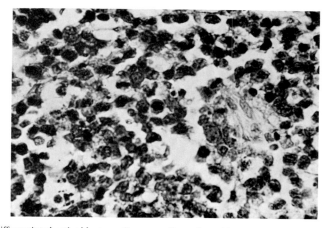

Fig. 9. Poorly differentiated retinoblastoma (hematoxylin-eosin, × 320).

TABLE 3.   METASTASES FROM RETINOBLASTOMA[a]

Focus	Reese (17 Cases)	Collected Cases (24)
Skull bones	9 (52.9%)	14 (58.3%)
Distal bones	9 (52.9%)	6 (25.0%)
Spinal cord	4 (23.5%)	6 (25.9%)
Lymph nodes	8 (47%)	8 (33.3%)
Viscera	8 (8%)	12 (50.0%)

[a] Modified from reference 19.

The degree of invasion of the optic nerve is an important prognostic indicator. If the tumor is small and the optic nerve head is not involved, the prognosis, as previously mentioned, is very favorable. If, however, there is extensive invasion of the optic nerve and orbit, the prognosis is considerably worse, particularly if the tumor extends beyond the line of surgical transection (Fig. 7). The surgeon performing enucleation should make an effort to obtain as long a section of optic nerve as possible. This therapy, along with earlier diagnosis, has contributed greatly to the much improved overall prognosis in these patients.[18]

A second important characteristic is the degree of cellular differentiation within the tumor. Well-differentiated tumors with numerous Flexner-Wintersteiner rosettes offer a very favorable prognosis (Fig. 8). Poorly differentiated tumors (Fig. 9) are somewhat more likely to spread. On the other hand, poorly differentiated tumors tend to respond better to radiotherapy, whereas well-differentiated tumors show resistance to radiation.[27]

Finally, the presence of choroidal invasion, once thought to be an indication of a poorer prognosis, has recently been shown to have little effect upon the overall prognosis.[28]

In summary, metastatic tumors to and from the eye may present numerous diagnostic and therapeutic problems to the clinician. Ophthalmologists working with such patients should be familiar with the clinical variations, diagnostic approaches, and metastatic patterns in such cases. Therapy, however, should be coordinated with other medical specialists, depending on the overall clinical pattern.

REFERENCES

1. Ferry, A. P., and Font, R. L.: Carcinoma Metastatic to the Eye and Orbit. *Arch. Ophthalmol.* **92**:276 (1974).
2. Shields, J. A., and Zimmerman, L. E.: Lesions Simulating Malignant Melanoma of the Posterior Uvea. *Arch. Ophthalmol.* **89**:466 (1973).
3. Shields, J. A., Rodrigues, M. M., Tasman, W. S., Annesley, W. H., Jr., and Sarin, L. K.: Lipofuscin Pigment over Benign and Malignant Choroidal Tumors. *Trans. Am. Acad. Ophthalmol. Otolaryngol.* (in press).
4. Coleman, D. J., Abramson, D. H., Jack, R. L., and Franzen, L. A.: Ultrasonic Diagnosis of Tumors of the Choroid. *Arch. Ophthalmol.* **91**:344 (1974).
5. Gass, J. D. M.: *Differential Diagnosis of Intraocular Tumors.* Mosby, St. Louis, 1974.

6. Hagler, W. S., Jarrett, W. H., II, and Humphrey, W. T.: The Radioactive Phosphorus Uptake Test in the Diagnosis of Uveal Melanoma. *Arch. Ophthalmol.* **83**:548 (1970).

7. Shields, J. A., Sarin, L. K., Federman, J. L., Mensheha Manhart, O., and Carmichael, P. L.: Surgical Approach to the ³²P Test for Posterior Uveal Melanomas. *Ophthalmol. Surg.* **5**:13 (1974).

8. Shields, J. A., Hagler, W. S., Federman, J. L., Jarrett, W. H., II, and Carmichael, P. L.: The Significance of the ³²P Test in the Diagnosis of Posterior Uveal Melanomas. *Trans. Am. Acad. Ophthalmol. Otolaryngol.* **79**:297 (1975).

9. Shields, J. A., Carmichael, P. L., Leonard, B. C., Federman, J. L., and Sarin, L. K.: The Radioactive Phosphorus Uptake Test in the Diagnosis of Ocular Tumors. In Croll M., Carmichael, P. L., Brady, L. W., and Wallner, R. J., Eds., *Nuclear Ophthalmology* (in press).

10. Shields, J. A., Carmichael, P. L., Leonard, B. C., Sarin, L. K., and Annesley, W. H., Jr.: The Accuracy of the ³²P Test for Ocular Melanomas. An Analysis of 300 Cases. I. Transconjunctival Technique. (Submitted for publication.)

11. Shields, J. A., Leonard, B. C., Carmichael, P. L., Federman, J. L., and McDonald, P. R.: The Accuracy of the ³²P Test for Ocular Melanomas. An Analysis of 300 Cases. II. Transcleral Technique. (Submitted for publication.)

12. Michelson, J. B., Felberg, N. T., Shields, J. A., and Foster, L.: Carcinoembryonic Antigen Positive Metastatic Adenocarcinoma to the Choroid. *Arch. Ophthalmol.* (in press).

13. Michelson, J. B., Felberg, N. T., and Shields, J. A.: Carcinoembryonic Antigen in the Evaluation of Intraocular Malignancies. *Arch. Ophthalmol.* (in press).

14. Ryan, S. J., Zimmerman, L. E., and King, F. M.: Reactive Lymphoid Hyperplasia; an Unusual Form of Intraocular Pseudotumor. *Trans. Am. Acad. Ophthalmol. Otolaryngol.* **76**:652 (1972).

15. Shields, J. A., and McDonald, P. R.: Improvements in the Diagnosis of Posterior Uveal Melanomas. *Trans. Am. Ophthalmol. Soc.* **71**:193 (1973); *Arch. Ophthalmol.* **92**:259 (1974).

16. Shields, J. A., McDonald, P. R., and Sarin, L. K.: Problems and Improvements in the Diagnosis of Posterior Uveal Melanomas. In Croll, M., Carmichael, P. L., Brady, L. W., and Wallner, R. W., Eds., *Nuclear Ophthalmology* (in press).

17. Jensen, O. A.: Malignant Melanomas of the Human Uvea. A Recent Follow-up of Cases in Denmark 1943–1952. *Acta. Ophthalmol.* **48**:1113 (1970).

18. Hogan, M. J., and Zimmerman, L. E.: *Ophthalmic Pathology; An Atlas and Textbook.* Saunders, Philadelphia, 1962.

19. Reese, A. B.: *Tumors of the Eye.* Harper and Row, New York, 1963.

20. Federman, J. L., Lewis, M. G., Clark, W. H., Egerer, I., and Sarin, L. K.: Tumor-associated Antibodies in the Serum of Ocular Melanoma Patients. *Trans. Am. Acad. Ophthalmol. Otolaryngol.* **78**:784 (1974).

21. Davidorf, F. H., and Lang, J. R.: The Natural History of Malignant Melanoma of the Choroid; Small Versus Large Tumors. *Trans. Am. Acad. Ophthalmol. Otolaryngol.* **79**:310 (1975).

22. Flocks, M., Gerende, J. H., and Zimmerman, L. E.: The Size and Shape of Malignant Melanoma of the Choroid and Ciliary Body in Relation to the Prognosis and Histologic Characteristics. *Trans. Am. Acad. Ophthalmol. Otolaryngol.* **59**:740 (1955).

23. Starr, H. J., and Zimmerman, L. E.: Extrascleral Extension and Orbital Recurrence of Malignant Melanoma of Choroid and Ciliary Body. *Int. Ophthalmol. Clin.* **2**:369 (1962).

24. Font, R. C., Spaulding, A. G., and Zimmerman, L. E.: Diffuse Malignant Melanoma of the Uveal Tract: A Clinicopathologic Report of 54 Cases. *Trans. Am. Acad. Ophthalmol. Otolaryngol.* **72**:877 (1968).

25. Jensen, O. A.: Malignant Melanomas of the Uvea in Denmark, 1943–1952. *Acta. Ophthalmol.* Suppl. 75 (1963).

26. Ellsworth, R. M.: The Practical Management of Retinoblastoma. *Trans. Am. Ophthalmol. Soc.* **67**:462 (1969).

27. Ts'o, M. O. M., Zimmerman, L. E., Fine, B. S., and Ellsworth, R. M.: A Cause of Radioresistance in Retinoblastoma; Photoreceptor Differentiation. *Trans. Am. Acad. Ophthalmol. Otolaryngol.* **74**:959 (1970).

28. Redler, L. D., and Ellsworth, R. M.: Prognostic Importance of Choroidal Invasion in Retinoblastoma. *Arch. Ophthalmol.* **90**:294 (1973).

Metastatic Tumors to and from the Eye: Radionuclidic Diagnosis

Robert J. Wallner, D.O.
Assistant Professor of Radiation Therapy
and Nuclear Medicine,
Hahnemann Medical College,
Philadelphia, Pennsylvania

Millard N. Croll, M.D.
Professor of Radiation Therapy
and Nuclear Medicine,
Director, Nuclear Medicine,
Hahnemann Medical College,
Philadelphia, Pennsylvania

Luther W. Brady, M.D.
Professor and Chairman,
Department of Radiation Therapy
and Nuclear Medicine,
Hahnemann Medical College,
Philadelphia, Pennsylvania

In 1970, Jensen[1] reviewed a series of 214 patients with primary malignant melanomas of the uvea. Of these patients, 53% died with evidence of metastatic disease at autopsy. Death is usually the result of blood-borne metastases, and although metastatic infiltration has been reported to almost every organ, the most frequent site of predilection is the liver. Often there is late occurrence of massive hepatic metastasis with complete absence of disease in other organs[2] (Fig. 1). The evaluation of metastatic liver disease is therefore important in determining patient prognosis.

In 1971, a study was performed at the M.D. Anderson Hospital and Tumor Institute[3] comparing the accuracy of scintigrams in the detection of metastatic liver disease with serum alkaline phosphotase (SAP) and bromsulphalein (BSP) determinations. It was concluded that, because it provided anatomical information, the liver scan was the superior study. Although the SAP and BSP determinations are as sensitive as the scan in indicating the presence of a pathological process, there is a higher percentage of false-positive results in patients with no anatomical evidence of metastatic disease. These false elevations may be related to systemic effects of cancer elsewhere in the body or to toxicity from therapeutic modalities. Liver scans yielded a lower false-positive rate and a higher correlation with the actual extent of hepatic involvement. It was concluded that the scintigram was the most reliable of the three tests for estimating the degree of improvement or progression of lesions under therapy.

Ferry and Font[4] in 1974 reported a clinicopathologic study of 227 cases of carcinoma metastatic to the eye and orbit in the registry of Ophthalmic Pathology at the Armed Forces Institute of Pathology. They concluded that, although malignant melanoma is generally regarded as the most common malignant intraocular tumor of adults, there is evidence to suggest that carcinoma metastatic to the eye is actually the more frequent occurrence. With few exceptions, tumors that metastasize to the eye or its adnexa are carcinoma.

Ocular/orbital metastases have a propensity to occur from specific organ systems. The breast is the most frequent primary site in the female, and the lung is the most frequent site in the male. Numerous radionuclides have demonstrated an affinity for localization in breast carcinoma including blood-pool agents, such as ^{99m}Tc-HSA[5] and ^{99m}Tc-pertechnetate,[6] and bone-seeking agents, including ^{67}Ga[7] and ^{87m}Sr.[8] Recently, another bone-seeking radionuclide, ^{99m}Tc-diphosphonate[9] has received considerable attention. Imaging with this compound permits examination of the breast in conjunction with a search for the presence of metastatic skeletal disease. Unfortunately, the breast scan is of limited clinical usefulness since metastatic ocular/orbital disease is usually a late presentation in patients with known primary breast carcinoma.

The ability to detect the primary site becomes more significant in the presence of ocular/orbital metastases from pulmonary carcinoma, since two-thirds of the metastatic lesions may be present prior to the detection of the primary tumor. This illustrates the well-known propensity of bronchogenic carcinoma to metastasize early, often before any other clinical evidence of the previously "silent" primary neoplasm. ^{67}Ga is a radionuclide with known tumor-localizing capabilities demonstrating a high affinity for pulmonary carcinoma (Fig. 2 a, b). ^{67}Ga also demonstrates significant localization in renal cell carcinoma (Fig. 3). The renal lesion is the only other primary neoplasm exhibiting such a striking tendency for manifesting ocular/orbital metastasis prior to the detection of the primary lesion. Whole body scans permit simultaneous localization of both osseous and extraosseous metastatic disease. Renal scans with other radionuclides (^{197}Hg, ^{99m}Tc-Sn-DTPA, and ^{99m}Tc glucoheptonate) are also of value in conjunction

162

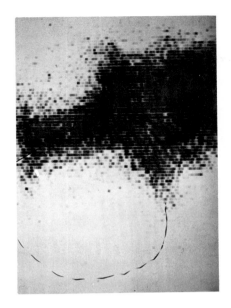

Fig. 1. ^{99m}Tc—sulfur colloid liver scan demonstrating massive replacement by metastatic melanoma.

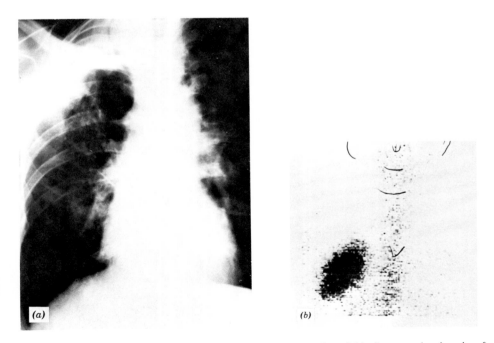

Fig. 2. (a) Chest x-ray revealing a mass density in the right upper lung field adjacent to the pleural surface. (b) ^{67}Ga localization in histologically proven oat-cell carcinoma.

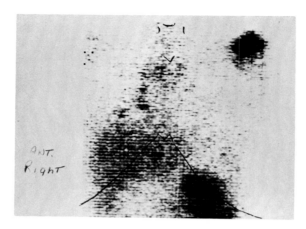

Fig. 3. [67]Ga localization in a left renal cell carcinoma with demonstration of metastatic lesions in the left shoulder, hilar and mediastinal lymph nodes and nodules in the right lower lung field.

with ^{99m}Tc-pertechnetate flow studies in demonstrating the presence of tumor neovascularity.

Ocular metastasis from primary malignant melanoma of the skin can occur,[10] albeit rare. The detection of generalized metastatic disease has clinical significance, since it is unusual for a patient with a primary uveal melanoma to present initially with clinical evidence of metastatic disease. It is essential to detect subclinical metastases to avoid inappropriate surgery and to permit initiation of palliative chemo-, immuno-, or radiation therapy. In a recent series,[11] 54% of sites of grossly evident or pathologically proven metastatic melanoma were detected by a routine ^{67}Ga scan. Radionuclide uptake was observed in both melanotic and amelanotic melanomas (Figs. 4 and 5). There was some

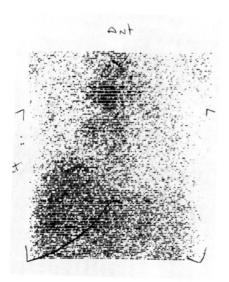

Fig. 4. [67]Ga localization in metastatic melanotic melanoma involving the right superior mediastinum.

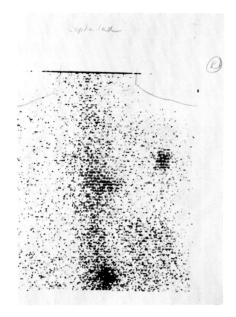

Fig. 5. ^{67}Ga localization in metastatic amelanotic melanoma involving right axillary, right hilar and right paravertebral lymph nodes.

variation in the ability to detect metastases in different organs. Bone lesions were most accurately visualized.

Lymph node metastases were detected in 60% of the known cases and constituted the most frequent site of involvement (following excision of the primary lesion). Skin and subcutaneous tumors had a detection rate of less than 50%, and no ocular melanomas were studied. Although ^{125}I-chloroquine is more specific for melanotic melanomas than ^{67}Ga citrate, it is less readily available, and its low energy gamma photons limit its usefulness to the detection of superficial lesions. ^{67}Ga can be detected in deep visceral metastases and permits the performance of whole body scanning procedures.

Metastatic tumors to the orbit from distant sites are unusual. The most frequent

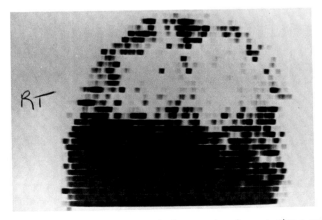

Fig. 6. Conventional anterior ^{99m}Tc-pertechnetate brain scan view demonstrating a unilateral increase in activity within the right orbit secondary to metastatic breast carcinoma.

Fig. 7.   Intense ^{67}Ga localization in the right orbit secondary to retroorbital metastasis from a primary squamous cell carcinoma of the right eyelid.

primary neoplasms include carcinoma (especially mammary gland and bronchial tree), sarcoma, and neuroblastoma. The neuroblastoma of childhood is a functional tumor, and one of its metabolic products is cystathionine, which can be identified in the urine. This amino acid is normally synthesized from methionine with homocysteine as an intermediate product. By labeling the basic amino acid methionine with selenium-75, it may be possible to demonstrate radionuclide localization in the primary or metastatic orbital tumor if cystathionine is being elaborated as a metabolic product.[12]

The presence of orbital metastatic disease may be detected by routine ^{99m}TcO$_4$ brain scans utilizing optimal technique and the conventional one-quarter axial anterior scan

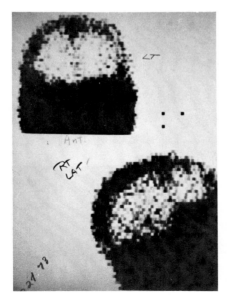

Fig. 8. ^{99m}Tc-pertechnetate brain scan revealing increased isotope localization within the left orbit with extension into the subfrontal region in the anterior view. Note the asymmetric peripheral increase in isotope localization in the right skull, which proved to be a metastatic lesion confirmed in the lateral projection.

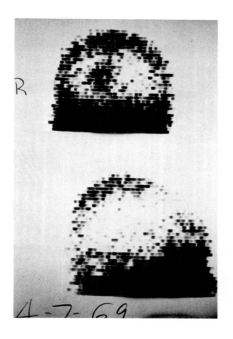

Fig. 9. Breast carcinoma metastatic to the right orbit with an additional intracranial metastatic lesion visualized by conventional anterior and lateral brain scans.

with the canthomeatal line perpendicular to the detector surface. However, maximal orbital visualization will be obtained employing the *en face* or direct anterior scan with 15–20° cephalad angulation of the canthomeatal line.[13] This view serves to elevate orbital activity above the level of background activity in the base of the skull. The presence of orbital metastasis is indicated by a unilateral increase in activity (usually representing an increase in vascularity or extracellular fluid) (Fig. 6). [197]Hg exhibits tumor-localizing properties and provides less background activity in the region of the skull and orbits. [67]Ga may demonstrate the presence of retroorbital metastatic lesions (Fig. 7). [67]Ga may normally concentrate within the lacrimal glands, however, and this activity should not be misinterpreted as representing the presence of pathology.

Whenever orbital scanning is performed, the study should not be limited to the orbital area but extended to include the entire anterior view of the brain (Figs. 8 and 9). The demonstration of abnormal radionuclide localization intracranially or within the skull will tend to confirm the fact that abnormal intraorbital isotope localization represents secondary or metastatic disease rather than primary pathology. The use of bone-seeking radionuclides may also be of value.

In summary, radionuclide studies can be of considerable value in the detection and confirmation of the presence of metastatic disease to and from the eye.

REFERENCES

1. Jensen, O. A.: Malignant Melanomas of the Human Uvea. *Acta Ophthalmol.* **48:**1113–1128 (1970).

2. Hogan, M. J., and Zimmerman, L. E.: Tumors of the Uveal Tract-Malignant Melanoma. In *Ophthalmic Pathology.* Saunders, Philadelphia, 1962, 429.

3. Jhingran, S. G., Jordan, L., Jahns, M. F., and Haynie, T. P.: Liver Scintigrams Compared with Alkaline Phosphotase and BSP Determinations in the Detection of Metastatic Carcinoma. *J. Nucl. Med.* **21:**227–230 (1971).

4. Ferry, A. P., and Font, R. L.: Carcinoma Metastatic to the Eye and Orbit. *Arch. Ophthalmol.* **92:**276–286 (1974).

5. Bonte, F. J., Curry, R. S., III, Oelze, R. F., and Greenberg, H. A.: *Radioisotope Scanning of Tumors.* Grune and Stratton, New York, 1969, pp. 138–142.

6. Cancroft, E. T., and Goldsmith, S. J.: ^{99m}Tc Pertechnetate Scintigraphy As an Aid to the Diagnosis of Breast Masses. *Radiology* **106:**441–444 (1973).

7. Langhammer, H., Glaubitt, G., Grebe, S. F., Hampe, J. F., Haubold, V., Hor, G., et al: ^{67}Ga for Tumor Scanning. *J. Nucl. Med.* **13:**25–30 (1972).

8. Papavasiliou, C., Kostamis, P., Angelakis, P., and Constantinides, C.: 87m Sr in Extra-osseous Tumors. *J. Nucl. Med.* **12:**265–268 (1971).

9. Berg, F. R., Kalisher, L., Osmond, J. D., Pendergrass, H. P., and Potsaid, M. S.: ^{99m}Tc-Diphosphonate Concentration in Primary Breast Carcinoma. *Radiology* **109:**393–394 (1973).

10. Font, R. L., Naumann, G., and Zimmerman, L. E.: Primary Malignant Melanoma of the Skin Metastatic to the Eye and Orbit. *Am. J. Ophthalmol.* **63:**738–754 (1967).

11. Milder, M. S., Frankel, R. S., Bulkley, G. B., Ketcham, A. S., and Johnston, G. S.: ^{67}Ga Scintigraphy in Malignant Melanoma. *Cancer* **6:**1350–1355 (1973).

12. D'Angio, G. J., Loken, M., and Nesbit, M.: Uptake of Selenium-75 Methionine in Tumor Sites of Neuroblastoma Patients. *Ann. Radiol.* **14:**351–353 (1971).

13. Wilson, E. B., and Briggs, R. C.: Study of Orbital Region in Brain Scanning, Using En Face View. *Radiology* **92:**576–580 (1969).

The Orbit and Adnexae

DYNAMIC FUNCTION STUDIES

Amaurosis Fugax

Richard E. Goldberg, M.D.

Associate Surgeon,
Retina Service,
Wills Eye Hospital;
Clinical Associate Professor of Ophthalmology,
Thomas Jefferson University,
Philadelphia, Pennsylvania

In 1952, Fisher defined amaurosis fugax as "periodic blindness in which the principal derangement is an interruption of the retinal blood flow, usually of one eye only."[1] These monocular ischemic attacks integrate the disciplines of neurology, radiology, ophthalmology, and internal medicine. They deserve critical consideration as symptoms of a potentially crippling or even life-threatening aortocranial occlusive vascular process.

HISTORICAL INTRODUCTION

Ischemic cerebrovascular disease has long been recognized. It was called "apoplexy" by Galen (130–200 A.D.); described as "softening" in 1761 by Morgagni; and 70 years later, Abercrombie stated that it was an ischemic condition caused by narrowing of the arteries in the "immediate" vicinity of the cerebral lesion. Abercrombie also suggested that extracranial factors were important, but investigators generally cleaved to finding local causes for cerebral softening. Gradually, extracranial causes of cerebral infarction were considered in the early part of the twentieth century; in 1951, Fisher suggested that the internal carotid artery was an important cause of cerebral infarction.[2, 3] This entity was dramatically demonstrated angiographically by Sjögrist (1936) and Moniz and his colleagues (1937).

It is now fully recognized that stroke may be caused by both intracranial and extracranial vascular disease. In accordance with the vessel involved, specific neurological syndromes are established. This chapter discusses the extracranial vessels.

ANATOMY

On the right side, the major portion of the blood supply to the brain is initiated by the common brachiocephalic trunk of the aorta. This divides into the subclavian artery, which supplies the arm, and the common carotid artery, which sustains the head; on the left side, the subclavian and common carotid arteries orginate independently from the aortic arch. The common carotid arteries pass cranially in the anterolateral aspect of the neck and midcervically divide into an external and internal carotid artery. The latter is the major source of blood supply to the eye and the cerebral hemispheres.[2]

The internal carotid artery enters the skull through the carotid canal of the petrous bone, curves anteriorly, medially, and then posteriorly, to pierce the dura mater anterior to the clinoid process. At this point, the internal carotid artery gives off its first branch, the ophthalmic artery, and this vessel proceeds through the optic foramen. The central retinal artery is the first and one of the smallest branches of the ophthalmic artery. It proceeds for a short distance within the dural sheath of the optic nerve, but about 1.25 cm behind the eyeball, it pierces the nerve obliquely and runs forward in the center of its substance to the retina.[4] When the central retinal artery enters the retina, it divides into the retinal vessels which lose their elastic tissue. Each quadrant of the retina is supplied by a major artery and vein. These are termed supero- and inferotemporal and supero- and inferonasal vessels. Retinal arteries and veins divide by dichotomous and sidearm branching.

There are a variety of vascular patterns on the optic nerve head. These largely depend on the level at which the major vessels divide. The central retinal artery and its primary branches lie nasally to the central retinal veins in the nerve head.[5] In approximately 25% of humans, a cilioretinal artery bends around the temporal margin of the disc to supply a portion of the macula.[6] For our purposes the significance of the external carotid artery is the branches it provides for collateral circulation of the brain.

Amaurosis fugax (fleeting darkening or blindness) reflects occlusive disease of the carotid system. Thus we will simply note that the subclavian arteries also give rise to the vertebral arteries which unite to form the basilar artery, which supplies structures in the posterior portion of the cranial cavity. Other potential sources of blood to the brain arising from the subclavian include the thyrocervical trunk and costocervical trunk.

The circulus arteriosus cerebri or circle of Willis lies at the base of the brain and is theoretically capable of balancing the apportionment of blood to all parts of the cranial cavity. In the presence of either basilar or internal carotid artery occlusion, the posterior communicating arteries may become extremely important conduits for collateral blood flow. Of particular importance, if the internal carotid artery is occluded unilaterally, is the potential collateral circulation of the proximal portions of the anterior cerebral arteries and the anterior communicating. Morphological variations can compromise this service.[2] When internal carotid artery occlusion exists, the main extracranial sites of collateral circulation are anastomosis between the ophthalmic artery and branches of both the ipsilateral and contralateral external carotid arteries.[2]

The site most often involved by atherosclerosis in the cervical vessels is the carotid bifurcation.[7] This is usually at the level of C4 and C5 vertebrae. Particularly the origin of the internal carotid artery and that portion of the common carotid artery adjacent to the origin of the internal carotid may be stenotic. Approximately one-third of individuals with evidence of cerebral ischemia have stenosis in these locations and, fortunately, these sites are accessible to surgery.[2] Ocular symptoms are present in 65% of patients with carotid insufficiency.[8]

PATHOPHYSIOLOGY

Atherosclerosis is characterized by the presence of nodular, irregularly distributed, yellow, fatty plaques involving the intima of large and medium-sized arteries. Initially, there is an *abnormal infiltration of lipids* into the intimal cells followed by regression, no change, or progression to a fibrous plaque. The *fibrous plaque* may also regress, remain static, or develop into a complicated atheromatous lesion. This lesion is characterized by the occurrence of one or more events: hemorrhage into the plaque, subintimal necrosis, loss of intimal continuity, ulcer formation, or calcification. Loss of intimal continuity may lead to the development of a thrombus within the lumen of the artery. The thrombus may progress to occlusive thrombosis or may fragment to produce thrombotic embolization.

Complicated atheromatous lesions are those most frequently associated with marked stenosis of the arterial lumen. Hemorrhage into the intima from the vasa vasorum may increase the size of the lesion and narrow the lumen. Ulceration of a plaque may occur in association with subintimal hemorrhage or subintimal necrosis, and the contents of plaques may be discharged to produce distal emboli.[2]

Loss of continuity in the endothelial surface overlying an atheromatous plaque exposes collagen, which causes platelets to aggregate on the roughened surface. The platelets then release adenosine diphosphate, which results in further aggregation of the platelets and initiation of the coagulation mechanism. A fibrinoplatelet plug is formed, and friable fibrinoplatelet material may break off and embolize distally to the eye or

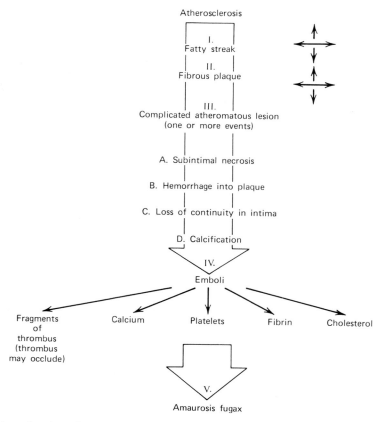

Fig. 1.   Atherosclerosis can lead to formation of microemboli which in turn can produce "amaurosis fugax."

brain.[2] The release of cholesterol, calcium, or fibrinoplatelet material into the circulation as a result of ulceration of a plaque in the carotid system or the occurrence of thrombotic embolization can produce amaurosis fugax (Fig. 1).

Atheromatosis is the usual cause of stenosis and occlusion of the carotid artery in middle-aged or older persons, but inflammation, trauma or congenital defects may be responsible in younger individuals. Carotid blood flow may also be reduced by fibromuscular dysplasia[9] and Takayasu disease (pulseless disease).[3]

AMAUROSIS FUGAX—CLINICAL FINDINGS

The clinical picture of internal carotid artery insufficiency is that of a monocular visual disturbance (amaurosis fugax) on the side of the lesion, separate from or coincident with motor and sensory changes on the contralateral side. The average age of patients with cerebral ischemic manifestations is 60 years, and men are affected twice as often as women. Hypertension is found in approximately half of these patients, and diabetes will coexist in 15%.[2] Statistically, there is evidence that about 50% of patients with intermittent insufficiency in the carotid or vestibular-basilar system will have a stroke within an average of 3 years, and the duration of the ischemia influences the pathologic changes occurring in the retina and brain. About 25% will continue to have episodes without stroke and the collateral circulation will lead to recovery of the other 25%.[10] Interestingly, if the internal carotid artery is involved, the time interval between the transient ischemic episode and a complete stroke is usually much shorter then if the vetebrobasilar system is the site of the lesion.[2]

Amaurosis fugax is a common symptom of carotid arterial insufficiency and occurs in about 40% of cases.[5] It consists of a sudden constriction of the visual field in one eye varying from the altitudinal anopsia to complete loss of vision followed by gradual return to normal within 4 to 5 minutes (at times somewhat longer) and usually not less than 2 minutes. It is often described as a visual loss simulating the lowering and then raising of a window shade or, less often, as a curtain moving from side to side.

During an "attack" of amaurosis fugax, the physician may note an absent pupillary light reflex, attenuated retinal arterioles, emboli, visual field defects (binocular if middle cerebral artery involved), "cloudy swelling," cotton-wool patches, venous stasis retinopathy, and Horner's syndrome. When present, obstruction of the central retina artery usually occurs at the lamina cribosa, and once occlusion occurs the involved retina becomes edematous, white, and opaque. The veins become darker and sludging is common. The narrowed arterioles also may sludge or show segmented arterial columns, and the uninvolved fovea transmits its normal red choroidal coloration. In branch artery obstructions, the retinal zone peripheral to the site of obstruction becomes infarcted.[5, 11]

Retinal arteriole pulsation occurs when the diastolic pressure is less then the intraocular pressure; thus, it may be noted in carotid stenosis, aortic arch disease, and aortic regurgitation. It may also be present with a normal arterial pressure if the intraocular pressure is sufficiently elevated (glaucoma).[11]

Other ocular responses to the reduced cervical blood supply include pain, photophobia, hyperemia (active congestion due to bypass by way of the external carotid artery), iritis, neovascularization of the iris surface, peripheral anterior synechiae, peripapillary neovascularization, choroidal atrophy, microaneurysms, ischemic neuropathy, cataract, and glaucoma, or hypotony.[12] Rarely, perforation of the globe can occur.[13]

One should suspect arterial insufficiency when the fundi demonstrate unilateral "diabetic retinopathy" (actually venous stasis secondary to arteriole underfilling) or asymmetric hypertensive retinopathy (better on the side with carotid disease).[5] This latter finding is not invariable, and the retinopathy can be more pronounced on the involved side.[14]

Ophthalmoscopy and auscultation with a bell stethoscope for evidence of a bruit over the common and internal carotid arteries (especially the bifurcation) are refreshingly elemental examination techniques. One-third to one-half occlusion is required to get an audible murmur. One should listen over the entire course of the carotid vessel with the patient both supine and sitting. It should be noted that many bruits are transmitted; should a bruit be heard over the globe of the eye, stenosis of the intracranial portion of the internal carotid artery (carotid siphon) may exist.

AMAUROSIS FUGAX—MICROEMBOLIC CAUSES

Ocularly, microemboli first impact at arteriolar bifurcations to cause blindness and then fragment and move peripherally, allowing return of circulation and sight. Three types of retinal microemboli, calcific—characteristically matte white and nonscintillating;

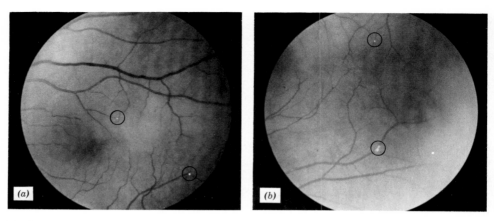

Fig. 2. (a) Yellowish, scintillating, multiple cholesterol-lipid microemboli (encircled) are noted in the retinal arterioles of this patient with a central retinal artery occlusion. (b) Cholesterol-lipid microemboli (encircled) noted in the retinal arterioles.

platelet-fibrin; and bright, yellowish, multiple cholesterol-lipid plaques (Fig. 2a,b), were mentioned earlier.

In an individual circumstance, embolization may be difficult to document because emboli that have become lodged in small vessels frequently fragment and travel more distally in the arteriole system, while others become lodged just posterior to the lamina cribosa and are invisible by ophthalmoscopy. The frequent origins of calcific emboli are vegetations from rheumatic valvalar disease of the heart and atheromatous plaques in the carotid artery or aorta. Microemboli of lipid material usually arise in an atheroma of a stenotic carotid artery. They may appear spontaneously, presumably from an internal ulceration of the artery, or may result from manipulation of the artery at the time of arteriography or endarterectomy or even trauma. Platelet-fibrinous microemboli occur with thrombocytosis as well as carotid disease. Myxomata of the heart are an occasional source of emboli.[11] Several cases of embolic occlusion of the central retinal artery have been reported clinically as secondary to these tumors.[15]

AMAUROSIS FUGAX—HYPOTENSIVE CAUSES

Transient retinal ischemic attacks may also be caused by critical hypotension in the terminal branches supplying the retina, brain, or both. Symptoms of hypotension appear first ocularly with a fall in cephalic blood pressure because the transmural pressure normally must be high in retinal vessels to counter the effect of intraocular pressure. Impaired flow in a stenotic carotid artery makes the ipsilateral retina more vulnerable to transient variations in systemic blood pressure (as precipitated by cardiac arrhythmia, postural hypotension, acute myocardial infarction, acute blood loss, Adams-Stokes syndrome and the use of certain medications). Elevated intraocular pressure may further jeopardize the retinal circulation in individuals with impaired flow in the internal carotid artery.[16]

Embolic phenomenon secondary to carotid artery disease and hypotensive episodes are currently accepted as causes of monocular blackouts. The concept of vasospasm in the distal arterial branches has been proposed but largely discarded (the retinal arteries have a dimunitive muscular coat). It may play a role during moments of sudden transient hypertension.

AMAUROSIS FUGAX—DIFFERENTIAL DIAGNOSIS

The differential diagnosis of amaurosis fugax includes monocular blackouts due to increases in orbital or ocular venous pressure (papilledema, retinal venous stasis or thrombosis, and glaucoma), cranial arteritis (and other causes of optic neuritis), migraine, severe anemia, retinal detachment, vitreous hemorrhage, and functional disorders.

The visual loss associated with embolic episodes usually lasts for several minutes, hypotensive episodes are usually briefer, and the monocular blackouts attributed to migraine routinely last for 10 to 20 minutes. Additionally, the scotoma in migraine is usually confined to one-half of the visual field and ranges from a small blind spot to total hemianopsia. Scintillating scotoma, fortification figures, as well as headaches, irritability, a family history, relation to certain foodstuffs, and nausea and vomiting may be present in individuals with migraine. Visual obscurations from papilledema or venous stasis are usually very brief.

Giant cell arteritis or cranial arteritis merits special consideration as it may be bilateral and cause catastrophic visual loss. This entity may occur more frequently in women than men and becomes more common after age 55. The temporal or occipital arteries are commonly involved, and ischemic optic neuropathy is responsible for the loss of acuity. There is often a history of headache, diplopia, polymyalgia rheumatica, anorexia, malaise, weight loss, and low-grade fever. Classically, the syndrome is associated with rather severe pain in the temporal or occipital regions and the vessels may be "ropy." Visual loss occurs in one or both eyes in 45 to 50% of the patients, and the ESR is elevated in 90% of cases. Although the visual loss is frequently abrupt, fleeting premonitory visual signs are noted. An afferent pupillary defect (Marcus Gunn pupil), dilatation and paralysis of the pupillary sphincter with or without signs of anterior segment necrosis, pallid edema of the disc with small nerve fiber layer hemorrhages, ischemic retinopathy, and central retinal artery occlusion are to be looked for. A temporal artery biopsy is contributory, and steroids must be initiated quickly.[17]

Ischemic optic neuropathy (vascular optic neuritis, opticomalacia) due to atheromatosis is another vasogenic process that merits mention. It should be differentiated from cranial arteritis. There is occlusion of the posterior ciliary arteries that supply the disc and usually no concurrent lesions in other locations of the central nervous system or pain are noted. Arterial narrowing, edema of the optic disc, with a few peripapillary hemorrhages followed by pallor and field defects are recorded. Anticoagulants and corticosteroids have been used without convincing results.[17]

OTHER METHODS OF EXAMINATION

Ophthalmodynamometry

The pressure in the retinal arteries may be easily measured by elevating the intraocular pressure through an external force applied to the sclera and simultaneously observing the retinal arteriole pulsations on the nerve head. The first induced pulsation corresponds to diastolic pressure, while the eventual elimination of pulsation and maintained collapse of the artery corresponds to systolic pressure.[11] Ophthalmodynamometry is valuable when positive. Unfortunately, incorrect technique, poor cooperation, false-negative results due to the external carotid collaterals supplying sufficient blood to the ophthalmic artery territory, or bilateral carotid disease all cause limitations.

Fluorescein Angiography

In the early 1960s, fluoroangiography was introduced as a dynamic method for visualizing the circulation in the posterior segment of the globe (Figs. 3a,b and 4a,b). Usually 5–10 cc of 10% fluorescein is injected into the antecubital vein. Fundus photographs taken in rapid sequence record the appearance and flow of fluorescein through the vessels. Normally, fluorescein enters the eye in 8 to 12 seconds after injection. As the choroid "lights up," or shortly thereafter (rarely before), fluorescein enters the retinal arteries and after a brief capillary transit time (about 2 seconds), it passes into the veins. A striking feature of the early venous phase is the lamination of the dye. Fluorescence clears from the retinal vessels in 5 to 10 minutes.[11]

CASE PRESENTATIONS

Two case presentations have been selected to illustrate many of the principles noted in this chapter.

Case 1.   A 55-year-old white female presented with transient obscurations of vision in the right eye. Visual acuity was 20/20-1 in the right eye and 20/20 in the left eye. Retinal hemorrhages secondary to venous stasis were noted near the equator of the right eye as well as in the retinal periphery. Interestingly, the central retinal vein was easily compressed. The right disc was hyperemic. The left fundus was normal.

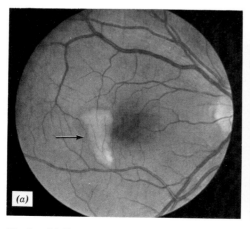 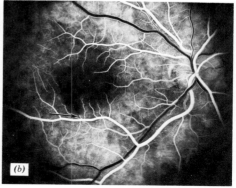

Fig. 3.   (a) Retinal photograph showing an area of ischemia or "cloudy swelling" (arrow) secondary to a small branch arteriole occlusion in the right eye of a young woman. (b) Fluorescein angiography dramatically demonstrates the blunted end of the occluded arteriole (arrow) below the right macula.

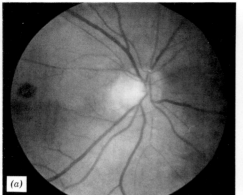 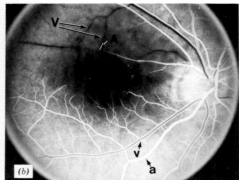

Fig. 4. (a) Superotemporal branch arteriole occlusion in the right eye of a patient with carotid stenosis. Note cloudy appearance of retina due to ischemia and presence of a small microembolus at 1 o'clock at the margin of the disc. (b) Fluorescein angiogram of fundus photograph noted in (a). At 16 seconds, one sees that the superotemporal retinal arteriole (O.D.) fills only approximately half way and the rest of the vessel appears black due to the absence of fluorescein (arrow-labeled "A."). The superotemporal retinal vein (arrows-labeled "V") servicing this area also fails to fluoresce due to underfilling of the accompanying arteriole. These superotemporal retinal vessels should be compared with the inferotemporal retinal artery (arrow-"a") and the inferotemporal retinal vein (arrow-"v"). The inferotemporal arteriole is filled and the inferotemporal retinal vein is in the normal laminar phase.

At this time, the fasting blood sugar was noted to be elevated; however, the asymmetry of the microangiopathy provoked continued critical observation rather then simple acceptance of glucose intolerance as the cause. Visual fields (tangent screen 3 mm white test object) were normal O.U. and the intraocular pressure was 18 O.D. and 19 O.S. (applanation). Fluorescein angiograms of the right eye failed to reveal any delay in the arm-to-retina circulation time.

Less then 3 months later, the blood pressure was elevated and a cotton-wool patch was noted temporal to the right disc. With the diagnosis of incipient vein occlusion, anticoagulation was initiated and carefully monitored. Five months later, the asymmetrical retinopathy remained unchanged, the veins were still easily compressed, and the anticoagulants were discontinued. The episodes of transient obscurations of vision in the right eye continued. At this time, fluorescein angiograms (O.D.) demonstrated some leakage of dye around the macula and this is compatible with stasis of the venules draining the macula (Fig. 5a,b).

Two months later, the visual acuity in the right eye dropped to 20/25-3 (pinhole no improvement). Ophthalmodynamometry (Bailliart) collapsed the right central retinal artery at a reading of five. Upon admission to the hospital, laboratory findings included the following: hemogram initially 14.8, 45% Hct, and 9,652 WBC with a normal differential. Later the Hb was 11, Hct 34% and 8,087 WBC's were noted with a shift to the left. Urinalysis was within normal limits. Screen I showed an LDH of 76 i.u., total bilirubin 1 mg%, SGOT 17 i.u. and alkaline phosphatase 27 i.u., uric acid 3.9 mg%, cholesterol 210 mg%, SGPT 29 i.u., total protein 6.8 gm%, albumin 3.8 gm%, globulin 3.0 gm%, a T_4 of 5.9 and calcium 8.5. Glucose was 118 mg%, BUN 11 mg%, sodium 140 mEq/l, potassium 5.8 mEq/l, chlorides 102 mEq/l and bicarbonate 23 mEq/l.

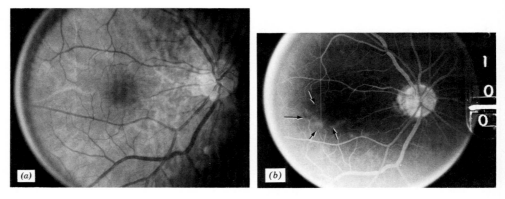

Fig. 5. (*a*) Fundus photograph of right eye with venous stasis retinopathy secondary to carotid insufficiency. This routine fundus photograph appears normal (compare with *b*). (*b*) The retina shows "wreath-like" staining around the macula (arrows) in the late sequences of fluorescein angiography (O.D.). This is compatible with stasis of the venules draining the macula.

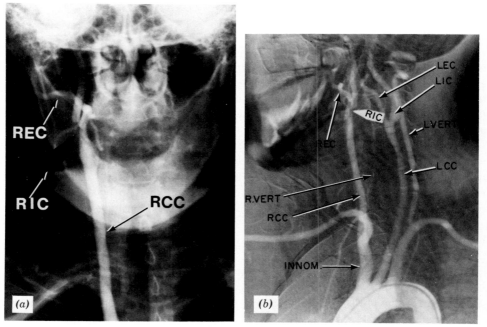

Fig. 6. (*a*) Demonstrates marked stenosis of the right internal carotid artery at its origin from the common carotid artery (arrow). (REC = right external carotid artery, RIC = right internal carotid artery, RCC = right common carotid artery.) (*b*) Angiography demonstrating marked stenosis of right internal carotid artery (white arrow). (R. Vert. = right vertebral artery, L. Vert. = left vertebral artery, RCC = right common carotid artery, LCC = left common carotid artery, RIC = right internal carotid artery, LIC = left internal carotid artery, REC = right external carotid artery, LEC = left external carotid artery, INNOM. = innominant artery.)

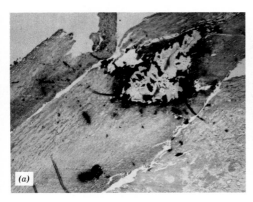
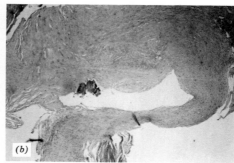

Fig. 7. (a) Pathology specimen from endarterectomy. Markedly thickened, hyalinized intimal tissue containing partly fragmented calcific deposit (above center) and capillary proliferation (right). (b) Pathology specimen from endarterectomy. Fibrous intimal plaque producing luminal compression (transport artifactual fragment within lumen). Cholesterol slits below lumen.

The electrocardiogram was normal on two occasions and the chest x-ray was normal except for slight thoracic scoliosis.

Angiography revealed marked stenosis of the right internal carotid artery at the origin from the common carotid artery (Fig. 6a,b). An endarterectomy was performed and since that time there have been no transient obscurations of the vision (Fig. 7a,b). The visual acuity is 20/20 O.U., visual fields are normal, spontaneous venous pulsations are present, all retinal hemorrhages have cleared (O.D.), and fluorescein angiograms are normal. Paresthesias and weakness of the left arm have cleared and there is no longer a systolic bruit over the right carotid. Seven months after the endarterectomy the ophthalmodynamometry was 50/35.

Case 2.   A 68-year-old white male noted a superior altitudinal defect in the left eye 6 days prior to admission. Four days later, he presented with an acuity of 20/25-2 in the

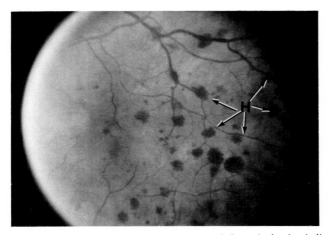

Fig. 8.   Blossom-shaped hemorrhages ("H" and arrows) around the retinal veins indicate the presence of venous stasis retinopathy due to arterial insufficiency (left eye).

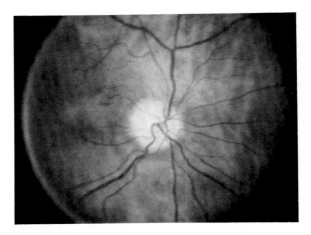

Fig. 9.   Early optic atrophy (left eye).

right eye and light perception with projection in the left eye. About 2½ years prior, he had experienced a transient loss of vision in the left eye, which took the form of a superior altitudinal field defect and lasted for 5 to 15 minutes before reverting to normal. Approximately 1½ years later, a similar situation occurred.

In the left eye the vision was light perception and ophthalmoscopy revealed an elevated blurred disc with segmentation and narrowing of the arterioles and concentric retinal convolutions temporal to the disc secondary to papilledema. The veins were engorged and irregular, and fundus photographs taken 1 month later documented blossom-shaped retinal hemorrhages due to venous stasis (Fig. 8). Optic atrophy was also recorded in the left eye at this time (Fig. 9). The anterior chamber demonstrated a slight flare and one plus cells. The intraocular pressure (applanation) was 19 and a Marcus Gunn pupil was present.

The right eye also showed blot and dot hemorrhages for almost 360 degrees near the ora serrata and some hemorrhages in the posterior pole (Fig. 10). The veins were

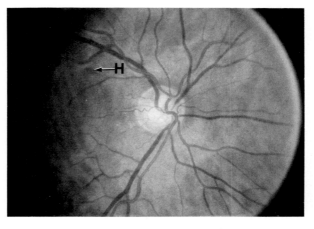

Fig. 10.   Superficial retinal hemorrhage ("H" and arrow) in the right fundus.

engorged and the central retinal artery pulsated when the globe was *gently* touched. The disc was normal, applanation pressure was 22, and the anterior chamber was clear.

A loud, harsh bruit was heard over the left carotid artery, but no bruit was present over the right carotid artery. There was a decrease in carotid pulsations bilaterally. No neurological deficits were noted.

The blood pressure was 170/110, the electrocardiogram was normal, and a 4-hour glucose tolerance test was normal. Urine protein analysis showed no abnormal protein. The electrophoretic pattern was normal. The LDH was 76 i.u., total bilirubin 1.2 mg%, SGOT 23 i.u., alkaline phosphatase 27 i.u., uric acid 4.2, cholesterol 300 mg%, SGPT 37 i.u., total protein 7.3 gm%, albumin 4.1 gm%, globulin 3.2 gm%, BUN 14 mg%, T_4 3.5 and calcium 9.6 mg%. Hemoglobin was 15, hematocrit 46%, 6,084 white count and normal differential. Sedimentation rate was 12, platelet count 274,000, L.E. Prep negative, and the initial prothrombin time was 100%.

Chest x-ray showed the heart was not enlarged, but the left ventricle was slightly prominent and aortic uncoiling was present. Hypertrophic changes involved the mid-

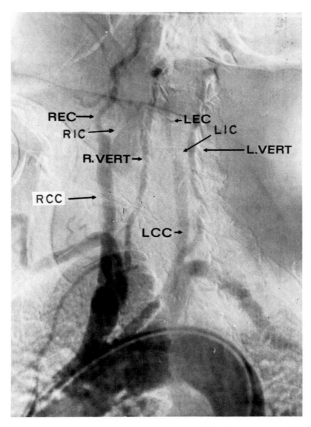

Fig. 11.   Aortic arch angiography demonstrating total occlusion of both internal carotid arteries at their point of origin from the common carotid. (REC = right external carotid, LEC = left external carotid, R. Vert. = right vertebral, L. Vert. = left vertebral, RCC = right common carotid, LCC = left common carotid, RIC = absence of right internal carotid artery which is completely occluded, LIC = absence of left internal carotid artery which is completely occluded.)

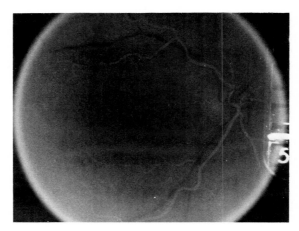

Fig. 12.   Fluorescein angiography documenting arm-to-retina circulation time of at least 25 seconds in the right eye (no sequences were available between 25 and 32 seconds).

thoracic spine, and the lung fields were clear. Aside from faint calcification, the skull x-ray was unremarkable. Cervical spine x-ray showed hypertrophic degenerative changes in the mid and lower portions of the cervical spine, with spur formation. There was marked narrowing of the third cervical interspace, and encroachment of several intervertebral formanina bilaterally.

Aortic arch angiography revealed total occlusion of both internal carotid arteries at the point of origin of the common carotid (Fig. 11). The external carotids were patent bilaterally and the common carotids appeared normal. Intracranially, there was good filling of the basillar and posterior cerebral arteries and extensive collateral vasculature over the surface of the brain. It was felt that the patient was receiving collateral blood

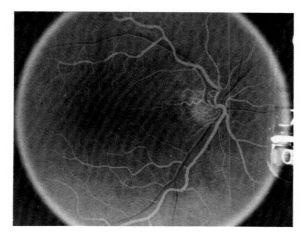

Fig. 13.   Delayed laminar venous phase (37 seconds) (right eye).

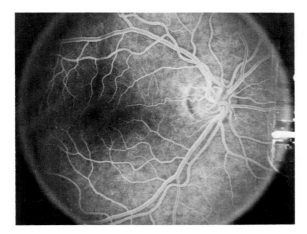

Fig. 14. Fluorescein angiography demonstrating presence of prolonged venous laminar phase 65 seconds after the dye injection (right eye).

supply to the portion of the brain normally serviced by both anterior and middle cerebral arteries via the external carotids, posterior cerebrals, and their collaterals. The technetium 99m pertechnetate cerebral blood flow study provided curves compatible with decreased perfusion to both hemispheres.

Initially, fluorescein angiography demonstrated an arm-to-retina circulation time of at least 25 seconds in the right eye (Fig. 12) (no sequences available between 25 to 32 seconds). Laminar flow was not seen in the central retinal vein until at least 5 seconds after the arteriole phase and it lasted 28 seconds (Figs. 13 and 14). Approximately 2 weeks after initiation of anticoagulants, the arm-to-retina circulation time had "improved" to 8.3 seconds (Fig. 15), but the appearance of the venous filling time

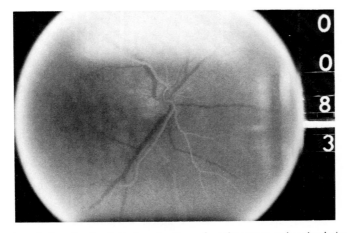

Fig. 15. Approximately 2 weeks after initiation of anticoagulant the arm-to-retina circulation time was noted to be 8.3 seconds in the right eye.

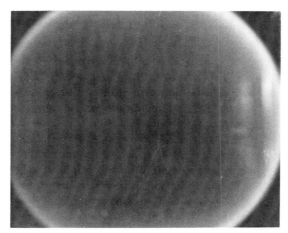

Fig. 16. One month after the initiation of anticoagulant therapy (and despite good control) the arm-to-retina circulation time had reverted to 23 seconds in the right eye.

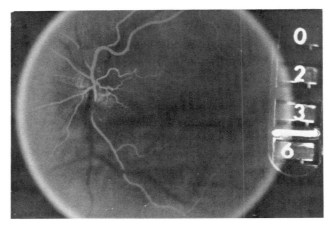

Fig. 17. Fluorescein angiography of the left fundus shows prolonged arm-to-retina circulation time (recorded between 19 and 23 seconds).

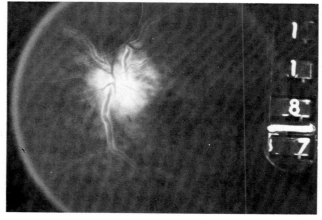

Fig. 18. Late in fluorescein sequence, angiogram demonstrates marked hyperfluorescence of the left optic disc secondary to ischemic neuropathy.

186

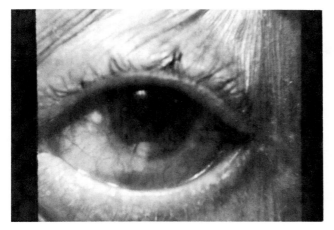

Fig. 19.   External photograph of left eye demonstrates marked conjunctival injection secondary to anterior segment ischemia.

remained delayed. One month later (despite anticoagulant therapy-prothrombin activity ranging from 22 to 34%), the arm-to-retina time had reverted to 23 seconds (Fig. 16).

Fluorescein angiograms of the left eye initially showed a prolonged arm-to-retina circulation time with the beginning of the arteriole phase recorded between 19 and 23 seconds (Fig. 17). Hyperfluorescence of the optic disc secondary to ischemic optic neuropathy was also recorded (Fig. 18).

Six weeks after the initial presentation, the visual acuity in the left eye decreased to no light perception, and 8 months after the first visit, this eye became painful. Three plus bulbar and ciliary conjunctival injection, corneal bedewing, a fixed dilated pupil, anterior nongranulomatous uveitis, severe neovascularization of the iris, and developing lens opacities were present (Fig. 19). The intraocular pressure was 28 mmHg. This anterior segment ischemia has been kept relatively asymptomatic with atropine and topical steroids. The visual acuity in O.D. remained at 20/20 throughout the 1 year follow-up.

SUMMARY

Because of the unique visibility of the fundus, clinical medicine has received many significant observations from ophthalmology. Amaurosis fugax provides another example of this productive kinship.

The role of cervical vascular disease in cerebrovascular disease is now well appreciated. The carotid vessels and retinal arterioles are part of an anatomic sequence and microemboli can travel this conduit. Resulting hypoxia may affect the anterior and posterior segments of the globe as well as the central nervous system. Significantly, the informed ophthalmologist is often in a position to discover evidence of occlusive vascular disease and initiate the appropriate evaluation.

ACKNOWLEDGMENTS

The author is grateful to Lester H. Wurtele, M.D., Department of Radiology and Nuclear Medicine of Holy Redeemer Hospital, Meadowbrook, Pa. for both performing and interpreting the angiography. The retinal photography done by Mr. Terrance Tomer, as well as the assistance of Mrs. Elaine DiMicco in typing several versions of the manuscript, is also greatly appreciated.

REFERENCES

1. Fisher, M.: Transient Monocular Blindness Associated with Hemiplegia. *Arch. Ophthalmol.* **47**:167 (1952).
2. Fields, W. S.: Aortocranial Occlusive Vascular Disease (Stroke). *Clinical Symposia* **26**:3–21 (1974).
3. Duke-Elder, S.: *System of Ophthalmology: Diseases of the Retina.* C. V. Mosby, St. Louis, 1967, pp. 357, 367–372.
4. Gray, H.: *Anatomy of the Human Body.* Lea & Febiger, New York, 1956, p. 640.
5. Wise, G., Dollery, C., Henkind, P.: *The Retinal Circulation.* Harper & Row, New York, 1971, pp. 20, 310, 311.
6. Hayreh, S. S.: The Cilio-Retinal Arteries. *Br. J. Ophthalmol.* **47**:71 (1963).
7. Gomensoro, J. B., Maslenkkov, V., Azambeya, Fields, W. S., and Lemak, N. A.: Joint Study of Extracranial Arterial Occlusion VIII. Clinical-Radiographic Correlation of Carotid Bifurcation Lesions in 177 Patients with Transient Cerebral Ischemic Attacks. *J.A.M.A.* **224**:985 (1973).
8. Hollenhorst, R. W.: The Ocular Manifestations of Internal Carotid Arterial Thrombosis, *Med. Clin. N. Am.* **44**:897 (1960).
9. Pollock, M., and Jackson, B. M.: Fibromuscular Dysplasia of the Carotid Arteries. *Neurology* **21**:1226–1230 (1971).
10. Hollenhorst, R. W.: In Smith, J. W., Ed., *Neuro-Ophthalmology*, Vol. II. C. V. Mosby Co., St. Louis, 1965, pp. 109–122.
11. Cogan, D. G.: Ophthalmic Manifestations of Systemic Vascular Disease. In Smith, L. S., Ed., *Major Problems in Internal Medicine,* Vol. III. Saunders, Philadelphia, 1974, pp. 23–28, 102–105, 120–124.
12. Michelson, P. E., Knox, D. L., and Green, W. R.: Ischemic Ocular Inflammation. *Arch. Ophthalmol.* **86**:274–280 (1971).
13. Clayman, H. M., Sandberg, J. S., and Altman, R. D.: Ocular Perforation in Pulseless Disease. In Glaser, J. S., and Smith, J. L., Eds., *Neuro-Ophthalmology Symposium,* Vol. 8, University of Miami. C. V. Mosby Co., St. Louis, 1975 (in preparation).
14. Miller, S. J. H.: Carotid Insufficiency. *Trans. Ophthalmol. Soc. U.K.* **80**:287 (1960).
15. Silverman, J., Olwin, J. S., and Grae Hinger, J. S.: Cardiac Myxomas with Systemic Embolization. Review of the Literature and Report of a Case. *Circulation* **26**:99 (1962).
16. Hoyt, W. F.: Retinal Ischemic Symptoms in Cardiovascular Diagnosis. *Postgrad. Med.* **52**:85 (1972).
17. Brude, R. M.: In Smith, J. L., and Glaser, J. S., Eds., *Neuro-Ophthalmology.* Symposium of the University of Miami and the Bascom Palmer Eye Institute, Vol. VII. C. V. Mosby Co., St. Louis, 1973, pp. 46–60.

Technetium 99m Cerebrovascular Flow Studies in Ophthalmology

Millard N. Croll, M.D.
Professor of Radiation Therapy
and Nuclear Medicine,
Director, Nuclear Medicine,
Hahnemann Medical College,
Philadelphia, Pennsylvania

Paul L. Carmichael, M.D.
Clinical Associate Professor
Department of Radiation Therapy
and Nuclear Medicine,
Hahnemann Medical College;
Assistant Surgeon, Retina Service,
Wills Eye Hospital,
Philadelphia, Pennsylvania

William Annesley, M.D.
Clinical Professor of Ophthalmology,
Thomas Jefferson University,
Wills Eye Hospital,
Philadelphia, Pennsylvania

Luther W. Brady, M.D.
Professor and Chairman,
Department of Radiation Therapy
and Nuclear Medicine,
Hahnemann Medical College,
Philadelphia, Pennsylvania

The ophthalmologist is often faced with the problem of further diagnostic testing in patients with transient ischemic attacks. The classical signs of these attacks are amaurosis fugax, unilateral optic atrophy with or without contralateral hemiplegia, systolic bruit over the course of the carotid artery in the neck, and fall of systolic pressure on the same side with ophthalmodynamometry.[1] Recently, retinal microaneurysms, retinal neovascularization, and rubeosis irides have been noted as additional ophthalmoscopic signs of possible carotid system disease.[2]

Ophthalmodynamometry is often used as a clinical test to determine central artery insufficiency.[3] Frequently, when a test is abnormal, or even when it is normal, one would like further confirmation of the clinical findings, but this usually involves carotid arteriography, with its known morbidity/mortality rate. In an effort to overcome this disadvantage, we investigated the use of radionuclide cerebrovascular flow studies in patients with suspected carotid artery insufficiency.[4]

MATERIALS AND METHODS

Studies were conducted in double blind fashion. The history, symptoms, and clinical findings were known only to the ophthalmologists, and the data were interpreted by the nuclear medicine physicians without history or clinical record.

A bolus of 15 mCi of ^{99m}Tc-pertechnetate is injected in the antecubital vein with a tourniquet in place. The cuff is rapidly released so that the intact bolus of technetium flows into the carotid circulation, having passed through the pulmonary circulation.[6] A multicrystal gamma camera* images the bolus of technetium passing through the carotid arteries and the cerebral hemispheres simultaneously on the right and the left sides. The images are stored on magnetic disk and tape. The tape is replayed after the study is completed, and specific anatomic areas of interest are identified for the computer. The data from the flagged sites are used to generate 100-point curves of the carotid and hemispheric flow patterns. A criterion of abnormality is that established by Mongeau[7] based on the time relationship as well as the amplitude of the derived curves. The times from cervical to maximal cerebral perfusion average 7 to 10 seconds and must not exceed 10 seconds, even in the elderly. Any delay of 2.5 seconds or more on one side relative to the other prior to establishing symmetry is considered abnormal.

The amplitude of the curves is compared by the formula: two times the square root of the maximum count of the higher curve is subtracted from the absolute count. The same technique is used for the lower curve, but the result is added to the absolute count. The resulting numbers from the high and low curves should overlap; if they do not, they are considered abnormal and asymmetrical. The transit time can be calculated by the first derivative method of Oldendorf.[2] Mongeau's studies have shown that values up to 9 seconds are normal and the values correlate well with the original findings of Oldendorf. Any discrepancy or more than 2 seconds between both sides is suspicious and more than 2.5 seconds between both sides is abnormal.

In analyzing the cervical artery curves, we find it necessary to tolerate a maximum of a 10% asymmetry. This is due to inclusion of the verterbral artery circulation as well as the carotids and could compensate for a partial internal carotid obstruction on one side. This has been evaluated by flagging of the area of the basilar artery. The results are listed in Table 1.

* Baird-Atomic, Inc., Bedford, Mass., model *System 70.*

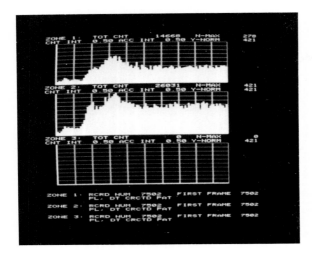

Fig. 1. Patient 22. Computer-generated curves of carotid flow reveal decreased flow through right side (upper) as compared to left carotid flow (lower).

CASE REPORTS

Patient 22.   A 61-year-old male who had three attacks of transient loss of vision on the right side within several months. The systolic ODM pressure was reduced on the right side. The clinical suspicion of insufficiency of the right carotid and right hemispheric circulation was confirmed by radionuclide diagnosis (Figs. 1 and 2).

Patient 2.   A 42-year-old male complained of flashing lights O.D. A diagnosis of impending central vein occlusion O.D. was made clinically. Radioisotope diagnosis confirmed the presence of right carotid and right hemispheric insufficiency (Figs. 3 and 4).

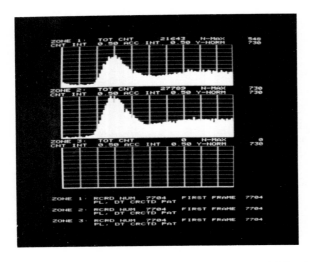

Fig. 2.   Decreased perfusion of the right hemisphere (upper) as compared with left hemisphere (lower).

TABLE 1

Patient Number	Symptoms and Signs	ODM	Clinical Diagnosis	Isotope Diagnosis
1	Left homonymous field defect Right CVA	25/50	Possible CVA due to right carotid block	Right hemispheric insufficiency Right carotid insufficiency
2	Flashing lights O.D.	60/40	Impending Central vein occlusion O.D.	Right hemispheric insufficiency
3	Flashing light O.S. Macular degeneration O.S.	60/40	Possible left carotid insufficiency	Left carotid insufficiency Left hemispheric insufficiency
4	Blurred vision O.S. Hollen-horst's placques O.U.	N/A	Possible bilateral carotid insufficiency	Right carotid insufficiency
5	Optic atrophy. Cataract O.S. blurred vision, flashing lights O.S.	65/35	Possible left carotid insufficiency	Left hemispheric insufficiency
6	Flashing lights O.U.	70/70	Possible cerebral arteriolarsclerosis	Left hemispheric insufficiency
7	Flashing lights, Central serous retinopathy O.S.	N.A.	Normal	Normal
8	Flashing lights O.S.	75/70	Possible left carotid insufficiency	Right carotid insufficiency Right hemispheric insufficiency
9	Transient visual loss O.S. Flashing lights O.D.	65/65	Normal	Normal
10	Amaurosis fugax: O.S.	60/60	Left carotid insufficiency	Left hemispheric insufficiency
11	Sudden visual loss O.S. Old visual loss O.D. Central vein occlusion O.D. Branch vein occlusion O.S.	N.A.	Possible right carotid insufficiency	Right carotid insufficiency Right hemispheric insufficiency
12	Light flashes O.D.	N.A.	Previous right carotid insufficiency. Endarterectomy successful	Normal
13	Light flashes, visual blur Arteriolar spasm and fullness veins O.D.	95/50	Impending central vein occlusion O.D.	Right carotid insufficiency Right hemispheric insufficiency
14	Light flashes O.D.	normal	Possible right carotid insufficiency	Normal

No.	Clinical findings	Value	Diagnosis	Interpretation
15	Sudden visual loss O.S.	75/75	Central artery occlusion O.S. Basilar artery insufficiency.	Normal
16	Flashing lights O.D. Fundi normal	65/70	Normal	Normal
17	Sudden visual loss: pain, redness O.S. Central vein occlusion. Absolute glaucoma	N.A.	Possible left carotid insufficiency	Left carotid insufficiency
18	Visual loss, optic atrophy O.D.	70/45	Possible right carotid insufficiency	Left carotid insufficiency
19	Blurring vision O.S.	N.A.	Normal	Normal
20	Vision blurred O.S. Central vein occlusion O.S.	N.A.	Possible left carotid insufficiency	Left hemispheric insufficiency
21	Double vision. Right CVA	N.A.	Possible left carotid insufficiency	Normal
22	Amaurosis fugax right	40/65	Possible right carotid insufficiency	Right hemispheric insufficiency Right carotid insufficiency
23	Peripheral retinal degeneration O.D.	N.A.	Normal	Normal
24	Ptosis; macular degeneration optic atrophy O.D.	70/40	Right sided insufficiency	Left carotid insufficiency Left hemispheric insufficiency
25	Headache left: macular degeneration	N.A.	Possible left carotid block	Normal
26	Decreasing vision; peripapillary atrophy: macular degeneration O.U.	N.A.	Possible cerebral arteriosclerosis	Left hemispheric insufficiency
27	Visual loss: optic atrophy O.S.	60/50	Possible left carotid block	Normal
28	Advanced senile macular degeneration bilateral. Left optic atrophy. Right-sided weakness of extremities	N.A.	Cerebral arteriosclerosis	Left hemispheric insufficiency
29	Flashing lights: bruit on right	30/60	Right carotid block	Right hemispheric insufficiency Right carotid insufficiency
30	Central vein occlusion O.D. Flashing lights	N.A.	Possible right carotid block	Normal

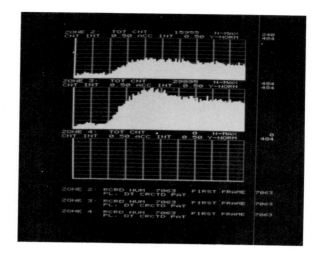

Fig. 3.   Patient 2. Decreased flow through right carotid artery (upper).

Patient 10.   A 62-year-old female complained of two attacks of fleeting visual loss within 2 months. Although ODM studies were equal in both eyes, the possibility of left-sided insufficiency was entertained clinically. The technetium studies indicated a left hemispheric insufficiency (Figs. 5 and 6).

Patient 1.   A 63-year-old male with a left homonymous field defect from a right CVA showed a definite right carotid and right hemispheric insufficiency on flow studies (Figs. 7 and 8).

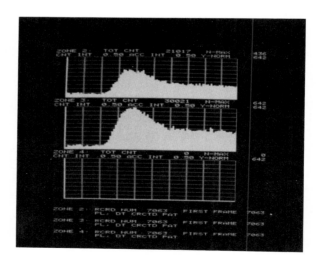

Fig. 4.   Patient 2. Decreased perfusion of the right hemisphere (upper).

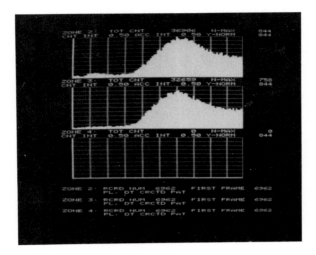

Fig. 5.   Patient 10. Flow through carotid arteries is symmetrical.

DISCUSSION

There were 30 patients studied in this series. Carotid or hemispheric insufficiency was diagnosed in 22 patients by radionuclide studies. Ophthalmodynamometry readings agreed with the technetium studies in 10 of 15 cases. Prediction of laterality of disease process agreed with the clinical findings in 19 cases. It is interesting to note that in central vein occlusion, of which there were 7 cases in the study, laterality of the disease process agreed with the site of intraocular involvement in 5 cases (Table 2).

Four patients in the series had arteriography performed. The results were unknown to the investigators until after the study had been completed. One patient had a previous carotid endarterectomy and the study was interpreted as normal. The other three cases agreed with the laterality of disease as confirmed by carotid angiography.

It should be noted that the radioisotopic technique for measuring cerebral blood flow presented here is not intended to yield measurement of regional brain blood flow as available from the Kety-Schmidt technique or the more popular tracer method utilizing

TABLE 2

Number of Cases	Procedure	Clinical Findings Signs and Symptoms	Cases in Agreement	
30	99mTc	Ipsilateral	19	(60%+)
30	99mTc	Bilateral	22	(70%+)
15	ODM	Ipsilateral	10	(60%+)
7	99mTc	C.V. occlusion Ipsilateral	5	
4	Arteriography	Ipsilateral	3	
6	99mTc	Mac. degeneration Ipsilateral	5	

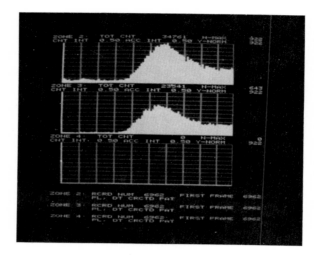

Fig. 6.   Patient 10. Hemispheric curves reveal decreased flow on left side (lower).

xenon-133 washout rate and relative chemical affinity. These techniques require injection into the internal carotid artery or selective intraarterial injection of the tracer.

Cerebral perfusion studies utilizing a bolus of technetium [99m] pertechnetate injected in the antecubital space and followed by subsequent imaging with a gamma camera yields very useful information. This is a comparative method in which the blood flow through the carotid artery and perfusion of the respective hemispheres is measured and compared to the flow on the opposite side.

The radioactive technetium tracer study is safer and more convenient than contrast radiography. The substance being used is a radionuclide and not contrast media. The site of injection is intravenous, usually in the antecubital vein, whereas in contrast ra-

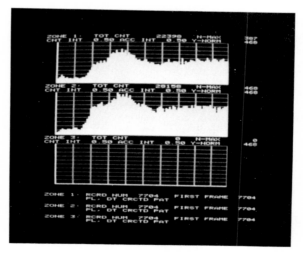

Fig. 7.   Patient 1. Decreased carotid flow right side (upper).

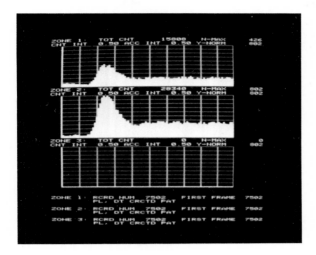

Fig. 8.   Patient 1. Decreased perfusion of the right hemisphere (upper).

diography a carotid artery injection is usually made. The study causes no morbidity or mortality.

SUMMARY

Technetium cerebrovascular flow studies can be a valuable adjunct to the ophthalmologist who suspects carotid system disease in his patient. The study can be performed with no anticipated untoward effects for the patient.

REFERENCES

1. Hedges, R.: Ophthalmoscopic Findings in Internal Carotid Artery Occlusion. *Bull. Johns Hopkins Hosp.* 3(2):89–97 (August 1962).

2. Kearn, T. P., and Hollenhorst, R. W.: Venous Stasis Retinopathy of Occlusive Disease of the Carotid Artery. *Proc. Staff Meet. Mayo Clin.* **38**:304–312 (1963).

3. Hollenhorst, R. W.: Ocular Manifestation of Insufficiency or Thrombosis of the Internal Carotid Artery. *Am. J. Ophthalmol.* **47**:753–767 (1959).

4. Hoefnagele, K. L. J.: Rubeosis of the Iris Associated with Occlusion of the Carotid Artery. *Ophthalmologia* **148**:196–200 (1964).

5. Grief, R. J., Wise, G., and Marty R.: Detection of Carotid Artery Obstruction by Intravenous Radionuclide Angiography. *Radiology* **97**:311–316 (November 1970).

6. Oldendorf, W. H.: Measurement of the Mean Transit Time of Cerebral Circulation by External Detection of an Intravenously Radioisotope. *J. Nucl. Med.* **3**:382 (1962).

7. Oldendorf, W. H., and Kitano, M.: Isotope Study of Brain Blood Turnover in Vascular Diseases. *Arch. Neurol. Chicago* **12**:30 (1965).

8. Mongeau, B.: Cerebral Blood Flow with the Multiple-Crystal Camera. In Croll, M. N., Brady, L. W., Tatem, H. R., and Honda, T., Eds., *Clinical Dynamic Function Studies with Radionuclides.* Appleton-Century Crofts, New York, 1972, p. 151.

Orbital Evaluation: The Role of Radionuclide Examination

Arthur S. Grove, M.D.
Instructor in Ophthalmology,
Harvard Medical School,
Boston, Massachusetts

Evaluation of the orbit is complicated by the wide variety of abnormalities which may involve the midfacial region. The most common orbital mass lesions which may cause exophthalmos are listed in Table 1.[1, 2, 3] It is important for physicians who deal with these abnormalities to be thoroughly familiar with the examinations available for orbital evaluation.[3] The most frequently used diagnostic aids are summarized in Table 2.

SPECIAL EXAMINATIONS

Ophthalmic Graves' disease is probably the most frequent cause of exophthalmos among adults.[4, 5] Screening evaluation of patients suspected of having this condition should include measurement of total thyroxine, free thyroxine, and total tri-iodothyronine. Some patients with Graves' disease may be hypothyroid or euthyroid with abnormal thyroid suppressibility. This may be investigated by use of tri-iodothyronine suppression test or by response to the administration of thyrotropin-releasing hormone. Antithyroid antibody abnormalities may help to establish the diagnosis of Graves' disease when other tests are equivocal. Enlarged extraocular muscles may be visualized on ultrasound B-scans and computerized tomographic scans. Technetium 99m pertechnetate may accumulate within inflamed muscles and gallium 67 citrate may be concentrated within the ipsilateral lacrimal gland of patients with orbital involvement from Graves' disease.

Plain film radiography has been reported to show abnormalities in more than one-third of patients whose exophthalmos is not due to Graves' disease. Radiologic linear or hypocycloidal tomography provides additional details of radiographic changes such as bone destruction. Xeroradiography may visualize calcifications that are not evident on plain radiographs. Since thermography measures body surface temperature patterns, it may be useful in the evaluation of vascular abnormalities.

Venography may determine the location and dimensions of some retrobulbar lesions, since the superior ophthalmic veins usually occupy symmetrical positions in each orbit. Positive contrast arteriography is most useful for the evaluation of intracranial abnor-

TABLE 1. MOST COMMON ORBITAL MASS LESIONS (IN APPROXIMATE ORDER OF FREQUENCY)[a]

1. Ophthalmic Graves' disease
2. Metastatic and secondary carcinoma
3. Hemangioma and lymphangioma
4. Idiopathic orbital inflammation ("pseudotumor")
5. Lymphoma
6. Neural tumors (including neurofibroma and optic nerve glioma)
7. Meningioma
8. Rhabdomyosarcoma
9. Lacrimal gland epithelial tumor
10. Dermoid and epidermoid

[a] Summarized and modified from references 1, 2, and 3.

From the Department of Ophthalmology, Harvard Medical School and Massachusetts Eye and Ear Infirmary, Boston. This work was supported in part by Research to Prevent Blindness, Inc. and Massachusetts Lions Eye Research.

TABLE 2.   SPECIAL EXAMINATIONS USED FOR THE EVALUATION OF
ORBITAL ABNORMALITIES[a]

Thyroid Function Tests
Plain film radiography
Radiographic tomography
Xeroradiography
Thermography
Venography
Arteriography
Orbitography
Ultrasonography
Computerized tomographic scanning
Radionuclide scanning
Miscellaneous[b]

[a] Summarized and modified from reference 3.
[b] Including IVP, CBC, urine examination, electron microscopy, tissue culture, and immuno-globulin studies.

malities, arteriovenous communications, and aneurysms. Since arteriography is more often associated with serious complications than other diagnostic procedures, it is not commonly used for orbital investigation. Orbitography is performed by injection of contrast materials directly into the retrobulbar muscle cone. Because it has sometimes been followed by vascular embolism and blindness, orbitography has been almost completely replaced by less dangerous examinations.

Ultrasonography permits the evaluation of both intraocular and orbital structures using high frequency sound waves. B-scan images are two dimensional and can be used to examine tissues tomographically (Fig. 1). Although the optic nerve and extraocular muscles can be visualized near the globe, lesions near the orbital apex and masses within or adjacent to the orbital walls may not be detected. A-scan ultrasonography is less useful for orbital investigation because the images are one-dimensional. Since Doppler ultrasonography measures relative velocity and direction of blood flow, it may be used to evaluate vascular abnormalities such as arteriovenous communications.

Computerized tomographic (CT) scanning is a technique of visualizing thin crosssections of the body with a narrow beam of roentgen rays which are received by a sensitive scintillation detector. Photon transmission measurements are converted into absorption coefficients which are displayed on an oscilloscope as tomographic images (Fig. 2). The tissue density of each point of these images can be numerically determined. The entire orbital contents may be visualized, together with the nasopharynx, the skull, and intracranial structures.[6]

Radionuclide orbital examinations utilize scintillation detectors which record the distribution of gamma-ray emitting radionuclides. With the use of scintillation cameras, radiopharmaceuticals (tracers) such as technetium 99m sodium pertechnetate can be rapidly followed through the cervical, orbital, and intracranial vessels (dynamic scintigraphy or radionuclide angiography).[7, 8, 9] A variety of radiopharmaceuticals have been used to anatomically visualize facial and cranial structures (static scintigraphy or radionuclide scanning). Since these tracers vary in the reliability with which they can be used to detect difference abnormalities, the localization and characterization of struc-

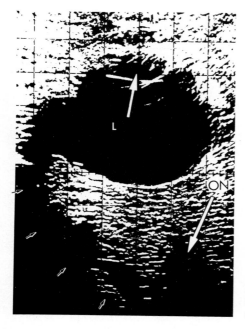

Fig. 1. Normal ultrasound B-scan showing optic nerve (ON), lens (L), and lateral rectus muscle (multiple small arrows) within retrobulbar fat.

tures can be most certain when scintigraphy is performed with multiple radionuclides.[8-11]

TECHNIQUE OF RADIONUCLIDE EXAMINATIONS

Localization of structures with radionuclides usually requires the accumulation of greater radioactivity within an organ or lesion than in adjacent tissues. Orbital details can be most clearly visualized by placing the patient's head in the frontal *en face* posi-

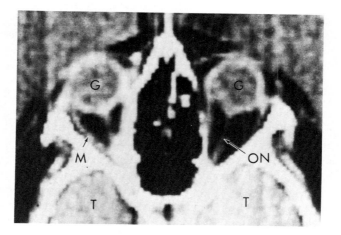

Fig. 2. Normal computerized tomographic (CT) scan showing both orbits. Globes (G), optic nerves (ON), extraocular muscles (M), and temporal lobes (T) visualized.

tion. The neck is extended so that the orbitomeatal line is 20° from a plane perpendicular to the face of the collimator (Fig. 3). The orbits are thereby interposed between the scintillation detector and the relatively low radioactivity within the cerebral hemispheres.

Oblique orbital views, which are analagous to radiographic optic foramen projections, are useful in accurately localizing and determining the anterior-posterior extent of orbital lesions. These views are obtained by rotating the patient's head slightly to the right and to the left of the frontal *en face* position (Fig. 4).

Total body or regional extracranial scans are sometimes useful in evaluating patients in whom orbital disease may be associated with systemic abnormalities. These studies are of special value when metastatic lesions or hematopoietic tumors such as lymphomas are suspected.

Since dynamic scintigraphy requires instantaneous monitoring of vascular flow, scintillation cameras must be used for these angiographic studies. Static radionuclide examinations can be performed with either cameras or rectilinear scanners. Although rectilinear scanners require a longer time to record images, they occasionally may show anatomic features in greater detail than is shown by scintillation cameras.

Dynamic scintigraphy is performed by first positioning the scintillation camera in front of the patient's head and then injecting 20 mCi of technetium 99m sodium pertechnetate as an intravenous bolus. The ^{99m}Tc rapidly flows through the heart and lungs and usually appears within the cervical carotid arteries within 5 seconds after injection. Subsequent passage through the orbital and intracranial vessels, and finally into the extravascular tissues (equilibration phage), is usually completed within 30 seconds after injection (Fig. 5).

Static scintigraphy is performed after an interval of several minutes to several days following injection of the radiopharmaceutical. The time between injection and scanning depends primarily upon the physical half-life of the radionuclide and upon the patient dose in millicuries. Studies using technetium 99m (6-hour physical half-life) are usually performed from 10 minutes to 6 hours after administration. Studies using longer-lived

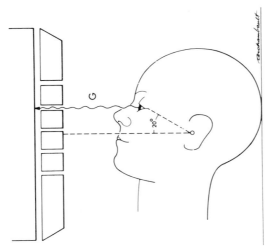

Fig. 3.   Diagrammatic representation of patient in frontal *en face* position. Gamma rays (G) which arise perpendicular to face of collimator strike scintillation detector.

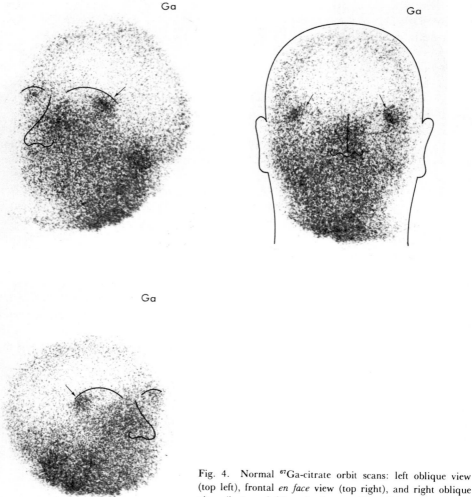

Fig. 4. Normal ^{67}Ga-citrate orbit scans: left oblique view (top left), frontal *en face* view (top right), and right oblique view (bottom left) each show radionuclide accumulation within lacrimal glands (arrows).

radionuclides such as gallium 67 (78-hour physical half-life) may be performed from 48 to 96 hours after administration.

By delaying examinations for some time after injection, radioactivity will often be increased in an abnormal lesion relative to surrounding back-ground activity. As a result, abnormalities may be detected with greater frequency using delayed studies than would be the case with earlier scintigraphy.[12, 13] When greater amounts of radioactivity are administered, the number of photons that are emitted are increased. Counting statistics and spatial resolution may therefore be improved.

SELECTION OF RADIOPHARMACEUTICALS

The distribution of radioactive tracers within the body is determined by their pharmacologic characteristics. The mechanisms of radiopharmaceutical localization differ depend-

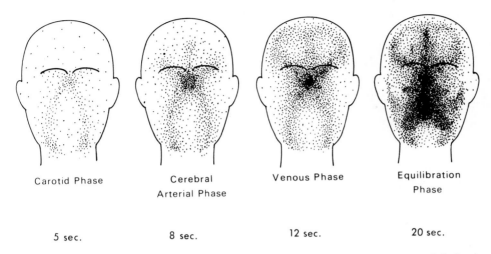

Carotid Phase

Cerebral
Arterial Phase

Venous Phase

Equilibration
Phase

5 sec.

8 sec.

12 sec.

20 sec.

Fig. 5.   Diagrammatic representation of normal dynamic scintigraphy (radionuclide angiography). Captions refer to phases of vascular transit and number of seconds after intravenous injection of TPT.

ing upon the histologic features of the involved tissues.[14] Tracers should be selected for orbital studies on the basis of their characteristics and the patient's clinical findings. Abnormalities can be diagnosed or characterized by dynamic scintigraphic flow patterns, by static scintigraphic distribution patterns, and by studying differential uptakes of multiple radiopharmaceuticals. Normal uptake patterns are considered "negative," while abnormal accumulation of radioactivity is usually graded as "weakly positive" or "strongly positive."

Because of commercial availability, patient safety, radiologic characteristics, and pharmacologic characteristics, most orbital studies at the Massachusetts Eye and Ear Infirmary and the Massachusetts General Hospital have been performed with several of four different tracers: technetium 99m sodium pertechnetate, gallium 67 citrate, technetium 99m diphosphonate, and mercury 197 chlormerodrin. The radionuclide physical characteristics are listed in Table 3, which also summarizes the usual adult doses and the time intervals between injection and static scintigraphy.

TABLE 3.   RADIOPHARMACEUTICALS USED FOR ORBITAL EVALUATION: PHYSICAL CHARACTERISTICS AND TECHNIQUES

Radiopharmaceutical	Physical Half-Life	Principal Gamma-Ray Energy	Usual Adult Dose	Usual Interval Between Injection and Static Scintigraphy
Technetium 99m sodium pertechnetate	6 hr	140 keV	20 mCi	10 min to 2 hr
Gallium 67 citrate	78 hr	93 keV	3 mCi	48 hr to 72 hr
Technetium 99m diphosphonate (Tc-1-hydroxy-ethylidene-1,1-disodium phosphonate	6 hr	140 keV	20 mCi	30 min to 6 hr
Mercury 197 chlormerodrin	65 hr	77 keV	1 mCi	2 hr

Technetium 99m sodium pertechnetate is the radiopharmaceutical which is used most commonly for both orbital and intracranial scintigraphy. Since ^{99m}Tc has a physical half-life of 6 hours and emits no beta radiation, large doses may be given to patients with only minimal radiation exposure. [99m]Tc can be visualized within blood vessels and accumulates in muscles, gastric mucosa, the large intestine, and the liver. It is also taken up by the thyroid, salivary, and lacrimal glands (Fig. 6).[15, 16, 17] The accumulation of ^{99m}Tc within abnormal tissues is relatively nonspecific, since the radiopharmaceutical localizes in most neoplastic, inflammatory, and vascular lesions.[8, 9, 11, 18]

Gallium 67 citrate gained clinical popularity because of its accumulation within tumors.[19] [67]Ga has a physical half-life of 78 hours and emits no beta radiation. Because of this long half-life scintigraphy may be delayed as long as 96 hours following injection. [67]Ga normally accumulates within the salivary and lacrimal glands (Fig. 4). Extracranial concentration is highest in the kidneys, adrenals, bone, spleen, and liver.[20, 21] Although ^{67}Ga accumulates in lymphomas and some other malignant tumors, it also localizes within granulomas and other inflammatory lesions.[22, 23]

Technetium 99m diphosphonate, which chemically is technetium-labeled 1-hydroxy-ethylidene-1, 1-disodium phosphonate, was synthesized for use as a skeletal-imaging radiopharmaceutical. The physical characteristics of technetium 99m have been described previously. The compound accumulates within normal bone and the kidneys.[24, 25] This tracer also localizes within soft tissue calcifications and a wide variety of bony lesions such as Paget's disease and malignancies.[25, 26]

Mercury 197 chlormerodrin has been used for orbital and intracranial scintigraphy because it accumulates within a wide variety of neoplasms.[8-11, 27, 28] Mercury 197 has a physical half-life of 65 hours, and emits both gamma and beta radiation. Because of these features and the fact that chlormerodrin accumulates within the kidneys, it is necessary to use relatively low doses of this tracer. When the usual adult dose of 1 mCi is used, the number of photons emitted is low and the statistical efficiency of the detector system is limited.

The results of orbital scanning with [203]Hg-chlormerodrin in combination with ^{99m}Tc have been previously reported.[8, 9, 11] It was shown that if orbital scans with both of these

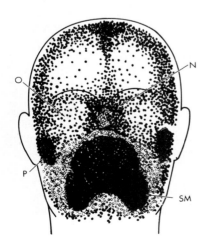

Fig. 6. Diagrammatic representation of normal frontal *en face* TPT orbit scan. Radionuclide visualized within parotid glands (P), submandibular glands (SM), oropharynx and nasopharynx (N). Orbits (O) contain relatively little radioactivity.

tracers were negative, then the presence of a neoplastic, inflammatory, or vascular lesion was unlikely. If scans with both of these tracers were strongly positive, then although a malignancy was likely to be present, lesions such as plexiform neurofibromas and cavernous hemangiomas might also be found. In this respect, multiple radionuclide scanning is a useful screening test for orbital malignancy, even though it must be remembered that false-negatives (rarely) and false-positives (more commonly) have been observed. The use of ^{203}Hg-chlormerodrin as a routine agent for orbital evaluation has recently been discontinued because of the necessarily low dose that can be safely administered, the poor counting statistics, and the relatively poor images. The remainder of this paper will therefore discuss the roles of ^{99m}Tc, ^{67}Ga, and ^{99m}Tc-diphosphonate in orbital diagnosis.

CLINICAL USES OF RADIONUCLIDE EXAMINATIONS

Noninvasive diagnostic techniques such as computerized tomographic (CT) scanning and B-scan ultrasonography anatomically visualize most orbital mass lesions. These and other nonradionuclide special examinations (Table 2) can be relied upon to localize most orbital and periorbital tumors. However, a significant number of abormalities may not be adequately visualized or characterized by the use of such examinations alone. In such instances, some of which are illustrated by the following examples, radionuclide examinations may play an important role.

Vascular Abnormalities

Carotid-cavernous sinus fistulas and arteriovenous malformations may be diagnosed by dynamic scintigraphy. Repeated radionuclide studies can be used to follow the course of these abnormalities without hazard to the patient (Fig. 7).

Ophthalmic Graves' Disease

Ophthalmic Graves' disease can be diagnosed by the recognition of characteristic clinical findings and abnormalities of thyroid function tests in most cases. Ultrasound examinations and CT scans sometimes demonstrate enlarged extraocular muscles or evidence of orbital inflammation. ^{99m}Tc usually accumulates in the pattern of a complete or partial "ring" surrounding the globe. ^{67}-Ga-citrate scans often show an increased accumulation of radioactivity within the ipsilateral lacrimal gland (Fig. 8).

Idiopathic Orbital Inflammation ("Pseudotumor")

Orbital inflammatory lesions of unknown etiology ("pseudotumors") are among the most difficult orbital abnormalities to diagnose. If such tumors are relatively circumscribed, both ^{99m}Tc and ^{67}Ga-citrate may be taken up as strongly positive focal accumulations of radioactivity (Fig. 9). If the inflammatory lesion is more diffuse, then a "ring" of uptake may be present on pertechnetate scans while ^{67}Ga-citrate more specifically outlines the tumor. Bony changes produced by such inflammatory lesions may be visualized on ^{99m}Tc-diphosphonate (Fig. 10).

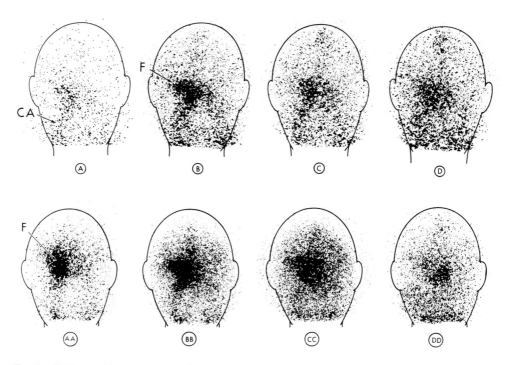

Fig. 7. Right carotid-cavernous sinus fistula studied by dynamic scintigraphy. Initial examination (A, B, C, D) shows greater activity in carotid artery (CA, arrow) on side of fistula (F, arrow) than on contralateral side. Repeated examination (AA, BB, CC, DD) 6 months later shows increased activity, suggesting progression in size of lesion. In both examinations abnormal activity declines rapidly and radionuclide distribution is almost symmetrical by equilibration phase (D and DD).

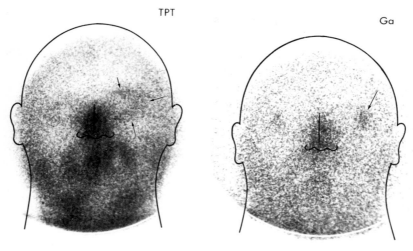

Fig. 8. Ophthalmic Graves' disease involving left orbit. TPT scan (left) shows "ring" of increased activity surrounding globe in area of extraocular muscles (arrows). ^{67}Ga-citrate scan (right) shows increased activity in area of ipsilateral lacrimal gland (arrow).

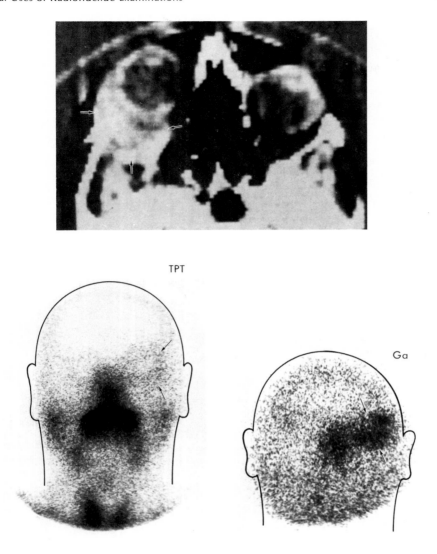

TPT

Ga

Fig. 9.   Idiopathic orbital inflammation ("pseudotumor") involving left orbit. Computerized tomographic CT scan (top) shows mass within left orbit (arrows) displacing eye forward. TPT scan (bottom left) shows focus of activity (arrows) plus associated inflammatory "ring". ⁶⁷Ga-citrate scan (bottom right) strongly positive in predominately lymphocytic lesion (arrows).

Hematopoietic Tumors

Hematopoietic tumors such as plasmacytomas and lymphomas may be discovered to be multifocal when total body or regional extracranial scans are combined with orbital examinations. ⁶⁷Ga-citrate scans are usually strongly positive in patients with such tumors (Fig. 11). ⁹⁹ᵐTc scans show less uptake than is evident with ⁶⁷Ga-citrate (Fig. 12).

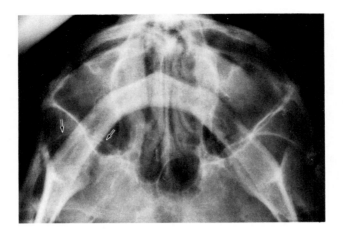

HEDSPA

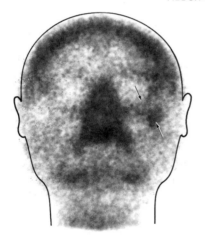

Fig. 10. Idiopathic orbital inflammation (same case as shown in Fig. 9). Basal radiograph (top) shows indistinct temporal fossa margin of right sphenoid (arrows). HEDSPA scan (bottom) shows increased activity in area of bony abnormality (arrows).

Meningioma

Meningiomas are characterized by some increased flow to the lesion during dynamic scintigraphy (Fig. 13). ^{99m}Tc static scintigraphy almost always shows a strongly positive accumulation of radioactivity in the area of the tumor. ^{67}Ga-citrate scans may be positive, but the uptake is less than is evident with ^{99m}Tc. Diphosphonate scans may be positive if bone is involved (Fig. 14). ^{197}Hg-chlormerodrin scans have previously been shown to be strongly positive in patients with meningiomas.[8]

In addition to the specific lesions that have been described, radionuclide scans may be used to determine the extent of infiltrative tumors such as plexiform neurofibromas.[11] The clinical course of proven abnormalities, including recurrence or persistence of tumors after treatment, may be followed by interval scintigraphy.

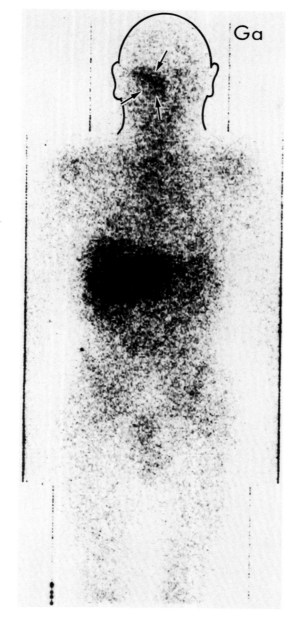

Fig. 11. Plasmacytoma involving right orbit (arrows) shown by ^{67}Ga-citrate scan. Total body examination also visualized thoracic and abdominal organs, but shows no abnormal extracranial accumulation of radio-nuclides.

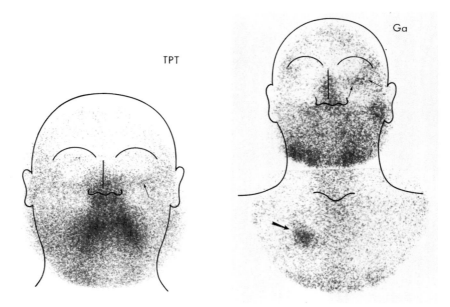

Fig. 12. Lymphoma involving left orbit. TPT scan (left) weakly positive (arrow). ^{67}Ga-citrate composite scan (right) shows strongly positive accumulation of radionuclide within left orbit (small arrows) and within chest wall to right of sternum (large arrow).

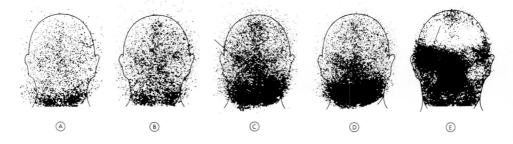

Fig. 13. Meningioma involving right orbit studied by dynamic scintigraphy (A, B, C, D) and 10 minutes later by static scintigraphy (E). Increased activity in area of right sphenoid begins during flow (C, arrow). Uptake progresses and becomes strongly positive in delayed examination (E, arrow).

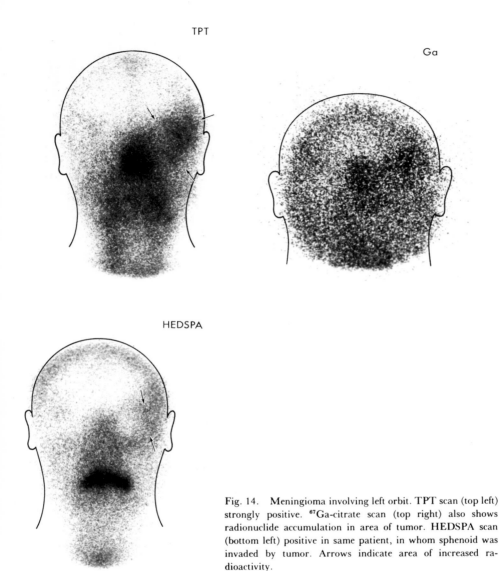

Fig. 14. Meningioma involving left orbit. TPT scan (top left) strongly positive. ⁶⁷Ga-citrate scan (top right) also shows radionuclide accumulation in area of tumor. HEDSPA scan (bottom left) positive in same patient, in whom sphenoid was invaded by tumor. Arrows indicate area of increased radioactivity.

SUMMARY

The special examinations that are most useful for orbital evaluation have been described. Those lesions that most commonly present as masses within the orbit have been listed. Radionuclide examinations can be performed for the evaluation of vascular abnormalities (dynamic scintigraphy or radionuclide angiography). Radionuclides can also be used to aid in the localization and characterization of solid lesions within the orbit (static scintigraphy or radionuclide scanning).

The frontal *en face* position and oblique views, together with total body or regional extracranial scans, may be useful in evaluating patients with orbital disease. Orbital studies were performed with technetium 99m sodium pertechnetate gallium 67 citrate, technetium 99m diphosphonate, and mercury 197 chlormerodrin. Some of the clinical uses of radionuclide examinations in the evaluation or orbital abnormalities have been presented.

ACKNOWLEDGMENTS

I would like to express my appreciation to Drs. Kenneth McKusick, Henry Pendergrass, and Majic Potsaid; and to the Division of Nuclear Medicine, Massachusetts General Hospital, for their advice and assistance in performing the studies described in this report.

REFERENCES

1. Reese, A. B.: Expanding Lesions of the Orbit. *Trans. Ophthalmol. Soc. U.K.* **91**:85–104 (1971).

2. Henderson, J. W., and Farrow, G. M.: Summary of 465 consecutive orbital tumors. In Henderson, J. W., Ed., *Orbital Tumors*. Saunders, Philadelphia, 1973, pp. 78–79.

3. Grove, A. S., Jr.: Evaluation of Exophthalmos. *N. Engl. J. Med.* **292**:1005–1013, (1975).

4. Moss, H. M.: Expanding Lesions of the Orbit. *Am. J. Ophthalmol.* **54**:761–770 (1962).

5. Reese, A. B.: A Series of 230 Consecutive Cases of Unilateral Expanding Lesions of the Orbit Studies Clinically. In *Tumors of the Eye,* 2nd ed. Harper & Rowe, New York, 1963, p. 533.

6. Grove, A. S., Jr., New, P.F.J., and Momose, K. J.: Computerized Tomographic (CT) Scanning for Orbital Evaluation. *Trans. Am. Acad. Ophthalmol. Otolaryngol.* **79**:137–149 (1975).

7. Grove, A. S., Jr., and Kotner, L. M., Jr.: Radionuclide Arteriography in Ophthalmology. *Arch. Ophthalmol.* **89**:13–17 (1973).

8. Grove, A. S., Jr.: Orbital Radionuclide Examinations. *Trans. Am. Acad. Ophthalmol. Otolaryngol.* **78**:587–598 (1974).

9. Grove, A. S., Jr.: Radionuclide Evaluation of the Orbit. In *Proceedings of the Second International Symposium on Orbital Disorders. Modern Problems Ophthalmology 14* S. Karger Basel, (in Press).

10. Di Chiro, G., Ashburn, W. L., and Grove, A. S., Jr.: Which Radioisotopes for Brain Scanning? *Neurology* **18**:225–236 (1968).

11. Grove, A. S., Jr., and Kotner, L. M., Jr.: Orbital Scanning with Multiple Radionuclides. *Arch. Ophthalmol.* **89**:301–305 (1973).

12. Gates, G. F., Dore, E. K., and Taplin, G. V.: Interval Brain Scanning with Sodium Pertechnetate Tc 99m for Tumor Detectability. *J. A. M. A.* **215**:85–88 (1971).

13. Ramsey, R. G., and Quinn, J. L., III: Comparison of Accuracy Between Initial and Delayed 99m Tc-Pertechnetate Brain Scans. *J. Nucl. Med.* **13**: 131–134 (1972).

14. Wagner, H. N., Jr.: Nuclear Medicine: Present and Future. *Radiology* **86**:601–614 (1966).

15. Webber, M. M.: Technetium 99m Normal Brain Scans and Their Anatomic Features. *Am. J. Roentgenol. Radium. Ther. Nucl. Med.* **94**:815–818 (1965).

16. Grove, A. S., Jr., and Di Chiro, G.: Salivary Gland Scanning with Technetium 99m Pertechnetate. *Am. J. Roentgenol. Radium. Ther. Nucl. Med.* **102**:109–116 (1968).

17. O'Nan, W. W., Wirtschafter, J. D., and Preston, D. F.: Sodium Pertechnetate Tc 99m in Lacrimal Secretion. *Arch. Ophthalmol.* **91**:187–189 (1974).

18. Mishkin, F. S., and Reese, I. C.: Tissue and Tumor Concentrations of Technetium 99m as Pertechnetate. *Am. J. Roentgenol Radium Ther. Nucl. Med.* **104**:145–149 (1968).

19. Edwards, C. L., and Hayes, R. L.: Tumor Scanning with [67]Ga Citrate. *J. Nucl. Med.* **10**:103–105 (1969).

20. Nelson, B., Hayes, R. L., Edwards, C. L., Kniseley, R. M., and Andrews, G. A.: Distribution of Gallium in Human Tissues after Intravenous Administration. *J. Nucl. Med.* **13**:92–100 (1972).

21. Silberstein, E. B., Kornblut, A., Shumrick, D. A., and Saenger, E. L.: [67]Ga as a Diagnostic Agent for the Detection of Head and Neck Tumors and Lymphoma. *Radiology* **110**:605–608 (1974).

22. Langhammer, H., Glaubitt, G., Grebe, S. F., Hampe, J. F., Haubold, U., Hör, G. et al: [67]Ga for Tumor Scanning. *J. Nucl. Med.* **13**: 25–30 (1972).

23. Higasi, T., Nakayama, Y., Murata, A., Nakamura, K., Sugiyama, M., Kawaguchi, T., and Suzuki, S.: Clinical Evaluation of ^{67}Ga-Citrate Scanning. *J. Nucl. Med.* **13**:196–201 (1972).

24. Castronovo, F. P., Jr., and Callahan, R. J.: New Bone Scanning Agent: 99m Tc-Labeled 1-Hydroxy-Ethylidene-1, 1-Disodium Phosphonate. *J. Nucl. Med.* **13**:823–827 (1972).

25. Pendergrass, H. P., Potsaid, M. S., and Castronovo, F. P., Jr.: The Clinical Use of 99m Tc-Disphosphonate (HEDSPA). *Radiology* **107**:557–562 (1973).

26. Miller, S. W., Castronovo, F. P., Jr., Pendergrass, H. P., and Potsaid, M. S.: Technetium 99m Labeled Diphosphonate Bone Scanning in Paget's Disease. *Am. J. Roentgenol. Radium Ther. Nucl. Med.* **121**:177–183 (1974).

27. Schlesinger, E. B., Trokel, S. L., and Bailey, S.: Radioactive Scanning in the Analysis of Unilateral Exophthalmos. *Trans Am. Acad. Ophthalmol. Otolaryngol.* **73**:1005–1012 (1969).

28. Trokel, S. L., Schlesinger, E. B., and Beaton, H.: Diagnosis of Orbital Tumors by Gamma-Ray Orbitography. *Am. J. Ophthalmol.* **74**:675–679 (1972).

Measurement of Relative Perfusion Distribution to Each Orbit Using Rapid Sequential Scintigraphy

John Weiter, M.D.
Research Associate,
Naval Medical Center,
Bethesda, Maryland

Rapid sequential scintigraphy is becoming widely accepted as a valuable noninvasive technique for the study of blood flow and tissue perfusion.[1, 2] The blood supply of a variety of organs has been evaluated by this means.[3-6] This dynamic technique has also been demonstrated to be of value in the detection of altered regional cerebral circulation.[7, 8, 9] In fact, some authors recommend its routine use as an integral part of all brain imaging procedures.[10]

Radioisotope imaging of orbital abnormalities has not received wide spread use because of poor resolution secondary to dense background activity. Kramer and Polcyn reported enhancement of orbital detail on brain scans by extension of the head.[11] This projects the orbits above the cavernous sinus and mucosal linings of the paranasal sinuses and in front of the brain, reducing background activity. Grove and Kotner recently reported favorable results in evaluating orbital abnormalities by supplementing static orbital scans with rapid sequential orbital scintigraphy.[12]

The purpose of this chapter is to emphasize the value of dynamic orbital radionuclide studies, using the recent modifications introduced by Schachar et al.[13] These modifications are twofold. The first is a pinhole collimator, which enlarges the radionuclide image of the orbits. The second is a magnetic tape playback with a region-of-interest counter, which allows measurement of counts per second from each orbit.

MATERIALS AND METHODS

In the preliminary studies performed at the University of Chicago Hospitals,[13] the equipment consisted of a scintillation camera* with the addition of a pinhole collimator and a data-store playback accessory. The results were printed by a high-speed digital counter. The pinhole collimator produced a magnified image of the radioactive pattern in the orbits.[14] The data-store playback accessory made it possible to continuously monitor the radioactivity in the orbits, and specific regions within each orbit.

Current studies performed at the National Naval Medical Center, Bethesda, Maryland, utilize two Anger-type scintillation cameras. Both are interfaced to a Medical Data Systems computer system capable of acquiring and processing data at framing rates of two per second in a 128×128 matrix.

As preparation, each patient received 1 g of sodium perchlorate ($NaClO_4$) orally, 30 minutes prior to testing to minimize the localization of the pertechnetate in the salivary glands, choroid plexus, thyroid gland, and stomach. The orbits were positioned 6–12 cm below the pinhole collimator with the head extended to obtain proper magnification[14] and to shift the blood-pool of the brain behind the orbits out of the region of interest to be counted[11] (Figs. 1 and 2). Sodium pertechnetate ^{99m}Tc was injected in an antecubital vein in a dose of 10–20 mCi, with the amount adjusted according to the weight of the patient. Scanning and recording began immediately after injection of the pertechnetate. The counts were accumulated and recorded for each second over a period of 16 seconds after injection. Compatible areas over both orbits were selected for analysis from the analyzer oscilloscope during data playback.

In this preliminary study of dynamic orbital scintigraphy, four patients with known abnormalities of orbital blood flow, along with two normal controls, are presented to demonstrate the value of this technique.

* Nuclear Chicago Pho/Gamma HP.

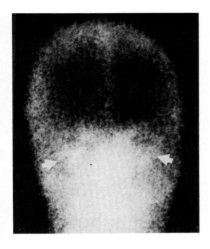

Fig. 1. Normal brain scan with routine anterior view. The orbits (arrows) are indistinct because of the superimposed high activity of the cavernous sinus and the mucosal linings of the paranasal sinuses.

RESULTS

The actual counts for each orbit reached a maximum of approximately 60 counts per second. To make the data easily comparable, they are expressed as percent of maximum counts per second. The percent standard deviation (% SD), obtained by the formula % SD = $\sqrt{N}/N \times 100$, where N is the number of counts per second,[15] was 13 percent.

Results from the examination of six representative patients are given in Table 1 and Figs. 3 to 7. In the normals, the perfusion distribution between the two orbits is very similar (Fig. 3). Enucleation of one eye resulted in no significant difference in perfusion distribution between the two orbits (Fig. 4). Exenteration, carotid compression, or sympathectomy resulted in measurable differences in perfusion distribution between the orbits (Figs. 5, 6, and 7).

The perfusion distribution curves for patients 2 to 5 demonstrate a secondary rise after the initial peak in activity. This was felt to represent an earlier perfusion of the orbits than of the cerebral hemispheres.

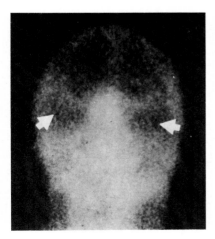

Fig. 2. Normal brain scan with the head extended. Views of the orbital areas (arrows) are enhanced.

TABLE

SUMMARY OF PATIENT DATA

Age, yr	Sex	Diagnosis	Difference in Blood Flow between Orbits	Standard Deviation
34	F	Normal	None	<1
53	M	Normal	None	<1
50	M	Right enucleation	None	<1
36	F	Right exenteration	Right <left	2
23	F	Silverstone clamp applied to the right carotid artery	Right <left	4
44	F	1. Right surgical sympathectomy	Right >left	>1
		2. At another time, right carotid manually compressed	Right <left	>1

DISCUSSION

Rapid sequential scintigraphy offers a simple, noninvasive technique for evaluating the flow of blood through vessels and organs. Sodium pertechnetate ^{99m}Tc is a safe, satisfactory radionuclide for the performance of these studies. When the studies are performed after prior perchlorate block of the glands, a 10 mCi dose of sodium pertechnetate ^{99m}Tc has been estimated to give a whole-body radiation exposure of 0.13 rads and 0.96 rads to the colon, the organ of maximum exposure.[16]

The complexity of the cerebral circulation and the limited resolution obtained has made interpretation of orbital perfusion studies more complicated. With modification of the standard view by extension of the head, enhancement of the orbital views can be achieved.[11] The present study demonstrates the value of two futher modifications in evaluating orbital blood flow, namely the use of a pinhole collimator and a magnetic tape playback with a region-of-interest counter.

This technique provides an index of variation in blood flow between the orbits of the same patient. It does not seem sensitive enough to measure changes in blood flow to the

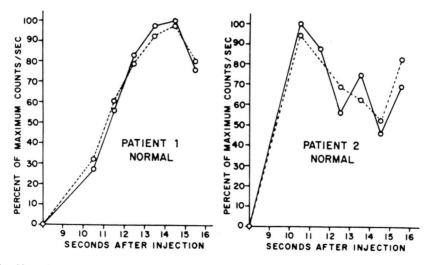

Fig. 3.   Normal rapid sequential orbital scintigraphy. Solid line—right orbit; broken line—left orbit. (From Schachar, R. A. et al.: Amer. J. Ophthalmol. 77:223–226, 1974)

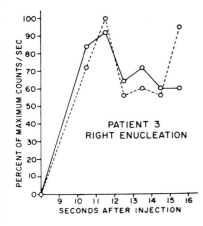

Fig. 4. Rapid sequential orbital scintigraphy following enucleation of right eye. Note no significant difference between
right orbit (solid line) and left orbit (broken line). (From
reference 13.)

eye, since there was no significant difference after enucleation. It does, however,
measure effects on orbital blood flow produced by exenteration, carotid compression, or
sympathectomy.

It is interesting to note that there was a 22% increase in blood flow to the orbit on the
side of the sympathectomy (Fig. 7). This corresponds with our measurements of ocular
blood flow in animals using radionuclide-labeled microspheres, in which we measured a
30% increase in blood flow to the sympathectomized side.[17]

An interesting preliminary observation is the shape of the perfusion distribution
curves. The secondary rise after the initial peak in activity was felt to represent an
earlier perfusion of the orbits than the cerebral hemispheres. This observation suggests
the possibility of having a method for differentially evaluating the ophthalmic artery circulation in relation to the middle cerebral artery circulation. The limited number of
patients studied to date preclude placing more emphasis on this finding.

This preliminary study was undertaken to determine the feasibility of orbital blood
flow evaluations using rapid sequential scintigraphy. The applicability of the technique
to large numbers was precluded at the time by the effort involved in handling the data.
With the rapid advance in solid-state technology in the past several years, most gamma

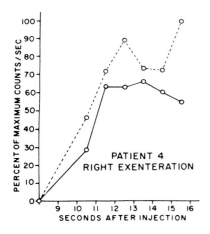

Fig. 5. Rapid sequential orbital scintigraphy following
exenteration of right orbit. A difference is noted between right
(solid line) and left (broken line) orbital areas. (From
reference 13.)

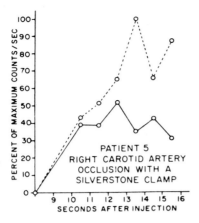

Fig. 6. Rapid sequential orbital scintigraphy following occulsion of the right carotid artery with a silverstone clamp. There is a significant difference between the right (solid line) and left (broken line) orbital areas. (From reference 13.)

scintillation cameras are now being interfaced with small general-purpose computers capable of acquiring, storing, and processing data. We are currently using a Medical Data Systems computer system at the Nuclear Medicine branch of the National Naval Medical Center, which allows good reproduction of information from the original in spatial resolution, data density, and data format. With this capability, we anticipate coupling dynamic orbital scintigraphy to static orbital imaging on a routine basis.[10]

SUMMARY

Rapid sequential scintigraphy is presented as an effective, noninvasive technique for study of the relative perfusion distribution to each orbit. Sodium pertechnetate ^{99m}Tc is

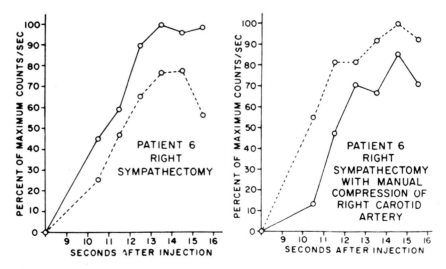

Fig. 7. Rapid sequential orbital scintigraphy. Solid line—right orbit; broken line—left orbit. The graph on the left demonstrates increased perfusion of the orbit after an ipsilateral sympathectomy, which can be significantly reduced by manual compression of the ipsilateral carotid artery (graph on the right). (From reference 13.)

injected intravenously, and its appearance in the orbits is monitored with a scintillation camera. The orbital evaluation is enhanced by extension of the head, use of a pinhole collimator for magnification, and a magnetic tape playback with a region-of-interest counter. The method is sufficiently sensitive to detect a decrease in blood flow to the orbits after carotid compression and exenteration, and an increase in blood flow after sympathectomy. The routine coupling of dynamic orbital scintigraphy to static orbital imaging on a routine basis is suggested.

ACKNOWLEDGMENTS

I should like to acknowledge with gratitude my colleagues Dr. Ronald Schachar and Dr. J. Terry Ernest, Department of Ophthalmology, University of Chicago, and Dr. Paul Hoffer and Ms. Violet Stark, Department of Radiology, University of Chicago, with whom this preliminary work was performed. My thanks are due Dr. Frederic Gerber, Nuclear Medicine branch of the National Naval Medical Center, for technical advice. This material has been published in part in the *American Journal of Ophthalmology*, volume 77, p. 223, 1974.

REFERENCES

1. Powell, M. R., and Anger, H. O.: Blood Flow Visualization with the Scintillation Camera. *J. Nucl. Med.* **7**:729–732 (1966).

2. Rosenthall, L.: Applications of the Gamma-Ray Scintillation Camera to Dynamic Studies in Man. *Radiology* **86**:634–639 (1966).

3. Polcyn, R. E., Poteshman, N. L., and Gottschalk, A.: Isotope Angiocardiography with Technetium-99m and the Scintillation Camera. *J. Nucl. Med.* **7**:374 (1966).

4. Kriss, J. P., Yeh, S., Farrer, P. A., and McKean, J.: Radioisotope Angiocardiography. *J. Nucl. Med.* **7**:367 (1966).

5. Powell, M. R., and Anger, H. O.: Triple Isotope Renal Evaluation with the Scintillation Camera. *J. Nucl. Med.* **7**:373 (1966).

6. Lavine, D. M., Fish, M. B., Pollycove, M., and Khentigan, A.: Rapid Scintiphotographic Placental Localizations utilizing Free 99m Tc Pertechnetate. *J. Nucl. Med.* **8**:773–784 (1967).

7. Ojemann, R. G., Hoop, B., Jr., Brownell, G. L., and Shea, W. H.: Extracranial Measurement of Regional Cerebral Circulation. *J. Nucl. Med.* **12**:532–539 (1971).

8. Moses, D. C., Nataranjan, T. K., Previosi, T. J., Udvarhelyi, G. B., and Wagner, H. N.: Quantitative Cerebral Circulation Studies with Sodium Pertechnetate. *J. Nucl. Med.* **14**:142–148 (1973).

9. Matin, P., Goodwin, D. A., and Nayyar, S. N.: Radionuclide Cerebral Angiography in Diagnosis and Evaluation of Carotid-Cavernous Fistula. *J. Nucl. Med.* **15**:1105–1109 (1974).

10. Cowan, R. J., Maynard, C. D., Meschan, I., Juneway, R., and Shigeno, K.: Value of the Routine Use of the Cerebral Dynamic Radioisotope Study. *Radiology* **107**:111–116 (1973).

11. Kramer, S. G., and Polcyn, R. E.: Extension of the Head for Orbital Scanning in Proptosis. *Am. J. Ophthalmol.* **69**:284–296 (1970).

12. Grove, Jr., A. S., and Kotner, L. M. Jr.: Radionuclide Arteriography in Ophthalmology. *Arch. Ophthalmol.* **89**:13–17 (1973).

13. Schachar, R. A., Weiter, J. J., Ernest, J. T., Stark, V., and Hoffer, P. B.: The measurement of Relative Blood Flow to Each Orbit by Dynamic Isotope Scanning Using Pertechnetate-99M. *Am. J. Ophthalmol.* **77**:223–226 (1974).

14. Heck, L. L., and Gottschalk, A.: Use of the Pinhole Collimator for Imaging the Posterior Fossa on Brain Scans. *Radiology* **101**:443–444 (1971).

15. Wagner, Jr., H., Walton, Jr., W. W., and Jacquez, J.: Statistics of Nuclear Measurements. In Wagner, H., Jr., Ed., *Principles of Nuclear Medicine.* Saunders, Philadelphia, 1968, p. 36.

16. Smith, E. M.: Internal Dose Calculation for 99m-Tc. *J. Nucl. Med.* **6:**231–251 (1965).

17. Weiter, J. J., Schachar, R. A., and Ernest, J. T.: Control of Ocular Blood Flow. 2. Effect of Sympathetic Tone. *Invest. Ophthalmol.* **12:**332 (1973).

Nuclear Dacrocystography

C. Craig Harris, M.S.
Associate Professor of Radiology,
Division of Nuclear Medicine,
Department of Radiology,
Duke University Medical Center,
Durham, North Carolina

Jack K. Goodrich, M.D.
Professor of Radiology,
Director, Division of Nuclear Medicine,
Department of Radiology,
Duke University Medical Center,
Durham, North Carolina

Arthur C. Chandler, M.D.
Associate Professor of Ophthalmology,
Associate in Anatomy,
Department of Ophthalmology,
Duke University Medical Center,
Durham, North Carolina

Jane K. Keiser, R.T.
Senior Nuclear Medicine Technologist,
Division of Nuclear Medicine,
Department of Radiology,
Duke University Medical Center,
Durham, North Carolina

Imaging procedures with radiopharmaceuticals, despite such disadvantages as nonspecificity of radiopharmaceuticals and statistical raggedness of the images, in some circumstances can produce diagnostic information more easily and effectively than previous methods. An outstanding example of such a study is the evaluation of lacrimal drainage by imaging the lacrimal drainage apparatus with a gamma scintillation camera fitted with a special pinhole collimator.

In 1972, Rossomondo and colleagues[1] introduced a technique whereby the passage of a minute quantity of radioactive liquid through the lacrimal drainage apparatus could be followed and recorded by imaging with a scintillation camera. They called the procedure "lacrimal microscintigraphy." "Micro" refers to the use of a "micropinhole" collimator, with an aperture of 0.043 in. (instead of the previous smallest, 0.177 in.) to obtain sufficient spatial resolution to resolve acceptably the images of the canaliculi. Chaudhuri et al, in reporting a comparison of the nuclear method with the radiographic procedure, referred to the study as "nuclear dacrocystography."[2] This procedure appears to be superior to all its predecessors in the quantity and quality of diagnostic information obtained, and in the lack of discomfort to the patient.

The procedure is useful (1) in the preoperative diagnosis of lacrimal drainage block, (2) for localizing the site of blockage or obstruction, and (3) in evaluating the success of corrective surgery.[2]

RELATIONSHIPS TO EARLIER PROCEDURES

A widely used test is the Jones fluorescein dye test;[3] it is simple but does not localize partial obstruction nor differentiate between inferior and superior canaliculi. The new test clearly resolves the canaliculi, requires no catheterization of the canaliculi, and demonstrates partial obstruction, provided only that an image is obtained at the proper time. The pressure transducer method of Callahan,[4] while capable of localizing obstruction, also requires catheterization.

A procedure widely used for some time for lacrimal drainage evaluation is radiographic contrast dacryocystography.[5] This is a definitive procedure, but requires local anaesthesia, dilation of the punctum, cannulation of the canaliculi, and injection of radiopaque dye under pressure which can cause false interpretation by opening physiologic obstructions or by creating false passages. Radiographs may show individual elements of the lacrimal drainage apparatus, but rarely show the entire passage; collections of the dye may be mistakenly interpreted as occlusion. Additionally, the procedure causes discomfort and leads to a radiation absorbed dose of 300–400 mrad *per AP skull roentgenogram*.[6] By comparison, the nuclear dacryocystogram involves a single drop into the eye and there is no internal sampling or catheterization. Moreover, the absorbed radiation dose to the eye is less than 10 mrad.[1, 2]

METHOD AND MATERIALS

Any scintillation camera equipped with a pinhole collimator may be used, provided a special 0.043-in. diameter pinhole* can be attached. A threaded-drive plunger assembly,† which facilitates the manual delivery of a single drop from a 25-gauge to 21-gauge needle on a disposable 1 ml tuberculin syringe, is also useful.

* D-I model 350 micropinhole for Searle scintillation camera. Dunn Instruments, San Francisco, California 94133.
† Dunn Instruments.

The administered material is a single drop of sodium pertechnetate ^{99m}Tc solution, containing about 100 μCi. This can be achieved by diluting, with normal sterile saline solution, eluted sodium pertechnetate ^{99m}Tc to 7.5 mCi/ml, and delivering with a 25-gauge needle (75 drops per ml). For a 21-gauge needle (60 drops per ml), the dilution should be made to 6 mCi/ml.

TECHNIQUE

1.   The patient is seated before the camera, with axis of the pinhole parallel to the floor and at eye level. The initial positioning is to demonstrate the position to the patient. The aperture of the collimator is aimed approximately .5 cm from the inner canthus. midway between the lid margins vertically, and at about 1 to 1.5 cm distance. The patient's nose may contact the lower side of the collimator for support; a rolled towel adds forehead support.

2.   The patient's head is tilted back until he is viewing the ceiling with both eyes open. It is important to image the normal eye (if any) first to establish positioning and to adjust imaging parameters. A single drop is delivered to the lateral aspect of the cornea. Usually the eyelids must be held open to avoid interference and to minimize splashes, as splashes and extra drops will invalidate the study.

3.   The patient is repositioned before the micropinhole and imaging and recording begun. With practice, this can be done in less than 4 seconds.

4.   To evaluate drainage, an initial image of 3000 counts is obtained; this requires 20 to 45 seconds. Succeeding 3000-count images are obtained and elapsed time recorded. The passage of the radioactivity and proper positioning of the patient is monitored by observation of a variable-persistence storage display oscilloscope. Delayed drainage is followed to 20 to 30 minutes.

5.   Just prior to termination of imaging, the patient is instructed to hold his nose and swallow, producing a negative pressure in the nasal cavity, a "negative Valsalva's maneuver." This is intended to promote lacrimal drainage into the nasal cavity, assuring patency of the orifices of the nasolacrimal ducts.

6.   After termination of imaging, the patient is moved away from the collimator, and both eyes are flushed with sterile physiologic saline. This reduces radiation absorbed dose in the eyes, particularly when drainage is impaired.

TYPICAL RESULTS

Case 1.   A 47-year-old white male had experienced an intermittent pain around the left eye for 10 to 12 years, which was relieved when he was able to express a lacrimal sac cast from the nasal pharynx. A lacrimal duct patency study (nuclear DCG) was performed. The right eye was studied first and drainage was normal. The left eye showed delayed, but effective drainage. Figure 1a shows the drainage from the normal right eye and the slower drainage from the left eye at comparable times (1 to 1.5 minutes). The difference in rate of clearance from the canaliculi is more evident later (4.5 to 5 minutes, Fig. 1b). Figure 2 shows the lacrimal drainage apparatus of both eyes after a "negative Valsalva's maneuver." Arrows indicate intranasal activity which assures patency of the orifices of both nasolacrimal ducts.

The problem was only intermittent, since it could be relieved by extrusion of the inspissated cast. Infection did not accompany the occlusion, therefore no intervention was attempted.

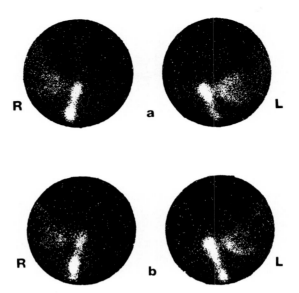

Fig. 1. Scintillation camera micropinhole images of lacrimal drainage apparatus, case 1. (*a*) Right and left drainage tracts are shown at 1 to 1.5 minutes after administration. (*b*) The tracts are shown at 4.5 to 5 minutes. Both sets of images show the relatively slower drainage of the left lacrimal drainage apparatus.

Case 2. A 40-year-old male had a long history of dacryostenosis with chronic epiphora and recurrent secondary conjunctivitis. A nuclear DCG was performed to determine if the stenosis was distal to the fundus of the lacrimal sac. Prior to this, several unsuccessful attempts to dilate and irrigate the lacrimal tract were made.

The left eye demonstrated normal drainage with much of the activity appearing within the nasolacrimal sac and duct by 3 minutes (Fig. 3*a*, L) and cleared from the canaliculi by 11 minutes (Fig. 3*b*, L). The right eye, in contrast, showed reasonably early entry into the lacrimal sac, but no drainage into the duct (Fig. 3, R). This finding was deemed consistent with the clinical diagnosis of stenosis of the right lacrimal duct. A dacryocystorhinostomy was performed. Upon follow-up examination, the patient appears to be doing well with no epiphora or conjunctivitis.

Case 3. A 24-year-old female experienced a sudden onset of dacryocystitis and increased epiphora. She was treated with ampicillin and hot compresses for 2 weeks.

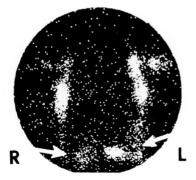

Fig. 2. Image of both lacrimal drainage tracts of the same patient in Fig. 1, after the conclusion of imaging the left tract, and after a "negative Valsalva's maneuver." Arrows denote intranasal activity which demonstrates the patency of the orifices of both nasal ducts.

The infection cleared, but when epiphora persisted, a nuclear DCG study was performed. The lacrimal drainage of the left eye was prompt and normal. Figure 4a shows a sequence of views; the radioactivity is shown mostly within the lacrimal sac and duct by picture 9 at about 3 minutes. The right eye, in contrast, at 5 minutes (Figure 4b, picture 10) shows accumulation in the lacrimal sac and proximal duct which persists to picture 13 at 15 minutes. The activity enters the nasal cavity only after a "negative Valsalva's maneuver" (picture 14). The final view (picture 15) shows both drainage tracts and dilatation of the right nasolacrimal duct. A residuum of activity is seen in the left nasolacrimal duct. The delay in lacrimal sac drainage without demonstrable obstruction led to continued conservative treatment and drainage returned.

Technical note: the patient's head should be comfortably restrained, as even slight patient motion can produce serious artifacts; see pictures 2, 7 and 9, Fig. 4b.

Case 4. A 34-year-old female gave a history of dacryocystitis and right-eye epiphora of 2 months duration. At examination, the right tear duct felt indurated. Apparently, however, gentamicin solution passed through the nasolacrimal duct as the patient re-marked of a characteristic taste in her mouth. A nuclear DCG was performed to determine the presence of obstruction by calculus or tumor and to assess function and appearance of the right lacrimal sac.

The normal left eye was studied first and showed prompt drainage (Fig. 5a). Drainage into the nasolacrimal duct was complete by about 7 minutes. A study of the right eye (which showed an overflow of radioactivity from tearing) gave evidence of partial obstruction just below the junction of the lacrimal sac and the nasolacrimal duct (Fig. 5b). In a repeat study with simultaneous administration in both eyes the point of narrowing and degree are well defined (lowest right picture, Fig. 5b).

Dilation was attempted; no stone was found and a conservative course was planned.

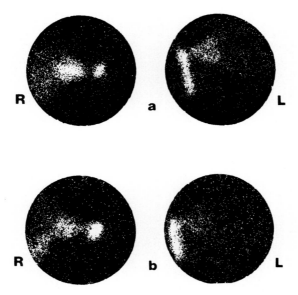

Fig. 3. Micropinhole images of the lacrimal drainage apparatus of case 2. Right and left tract images are shown at 3 minutes after administration at a, and at 11 minutes at b. The left eye demonstrates normal drainage; the right eye shows activity in the lacrimal sac, but no drainage.

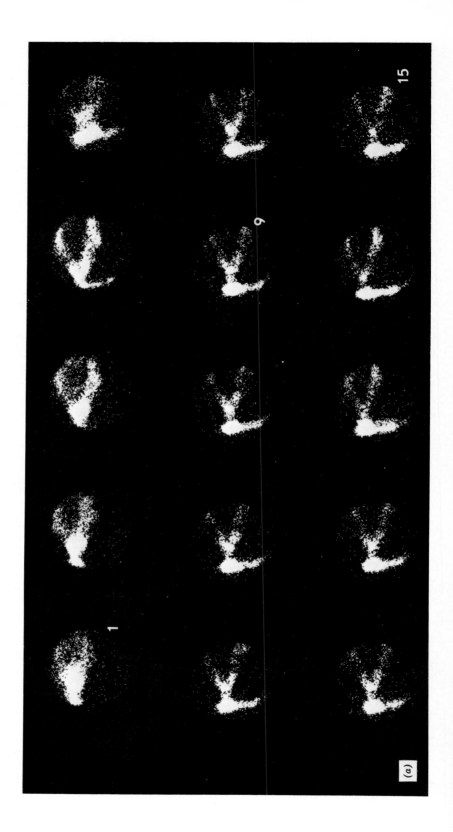

230

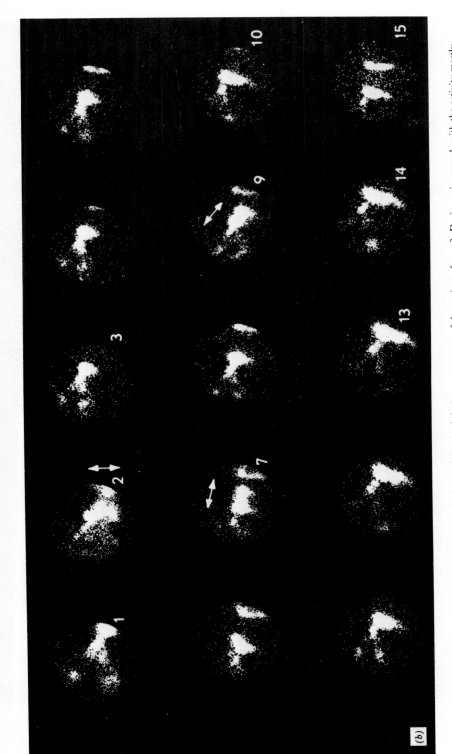

Fig. 4. (a) A 15-picture sequence of 3000-count images of the left lacrimal drainage apparatus of the patient of case 3. Drainage is normal, with the activity mostly within the lacrimal sac and duct by 3 minutes (picture 9). (b) A 14-picture sequence of the same patient, right eye. Activity is shown persisting in the lacrimal sac and duct through picture 13, entering the nasal cavity only after a "negative Valsalva's maneuver" (picture 14). Picture 15 shows both tracts and dilatation of the right nasolacrimal duct. Patient-motion artifacts are shown in pictures 2, 7, and 9.

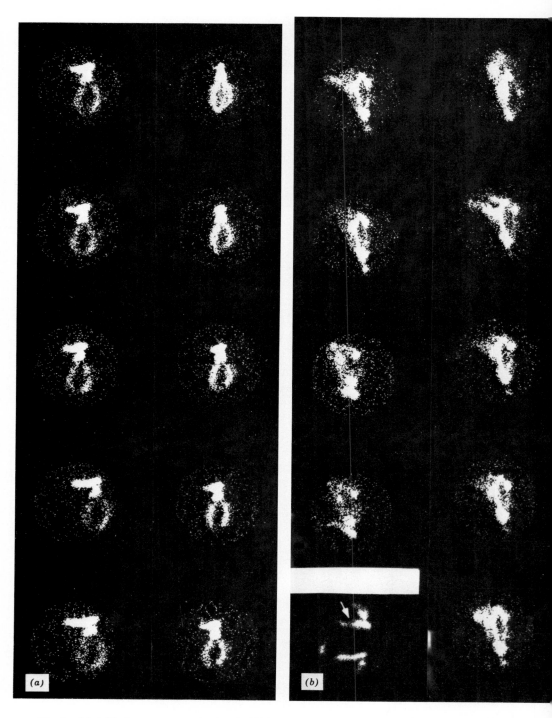

Fig. 5.   (a) A 10-picture sequence showing the left lacrimal drainage apparatus of the patient of case 4. (The sequence starts at the upper left and proceeds to the right; the lower right picture is the last in the sequence.) Drainage into the nasolacrimal duct was almost complete by about 7 minutes (last picture). (b) A 9-picture sequence, of the right eye of the same patient, in the same directions as Fig. 5a, followed at the lower right by a picture of both lacrimal drainage tracts after a second administration of radioactivity. Spread of activity due to tearing is evident. The sequence study indicates partial obstruction which is made more evident in the last picture (arrow).

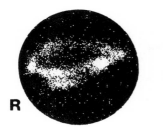 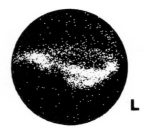

R   L

Fig. 6.   Images of right and left eyes of the patient of case 5. There is no evidence of entry of activity into the lacrimal sac of either eye.

Case 5.   A 46-year-old female gave a history of dacryocystitis of the left eye. Two dacryocystorhinostomies had been performed, but epiphora persisted. She noted also occasions of epiphora from the right eye as well. A nuclear DCG was performed to determine the anatomic level of obstruction in anticipation of further corrective surgery.

The study showed bilateral obstruction to lacrimal drainage between the common canaliculus[5] and the lacrimal sac of each eye (Fig. 6). This was further supported when cannulation and irrigation of the inferior canaliculus produced reflux through the superior canaliculus. The determination to install a Wadsworth-Chandler tube[7, 8] was made.

SUMMARY

Nuclear dacryocystography, or radionuclidic evaluation of lacrimal drainage by imaging, is a useful new procedure. It is uncomplicated, painless, and performed with readily available materials. The diagnostic value to the ophthalmologist is enhanced by the fact that the anatomy and physiology of the lacrimal drainage apparatus is not altered, thus providing a conservation approach for determination of treatment. The use of contrast radiography may be reserved for the visualization of ultrafine detail or intraluminal masses.[5]

ACKNOWLEDGMENTS

The authors express their gratitude to Mrs. Sharon Hamblen of the Division of Nuclear Medicine for her efforts in instituting and standardizing the procedure in our institution. The authors also thank Drs. Joseph A. C. Wadsworth, W. Banks Anderson, Jr., and Jack D. Davidson for consultations and discussions on the case reports.

REFERENCES

1.   Rossomondo, R. M., Carolton, W. H. Trueblood, J. H., and Thomas, R. P.: A New Method of Evaluating Lacrimal Drainage. *Arch. Ophthalmol.* **88**:523 (1972).

1.   Chaudhuri, T. K., Saparoff, G. R., Dolan, K. D., and Chaudhuri, T. K.: A Comparative Study of Contrast Dacryocystogram and Nuclear Dacryocystogram. *J. Nucl. Med.* **16**:605 (1975).

3.   Jones, L. T., and Boyden, G. L.: *Otolaryngology,* Vol. 3. W. F. Prior Co., Hagerstown, Md., 1955.

4.   Callahan, W. P., Forbath, P. G., and Besser, W. D. S.: A Method of Determining the Patency of the Nasolacrimal Apparatus, *Am. J. Ophthalmol.* **60**:475 (1965).

5.   Pettit, T. H., and Coin, C. G.: Dacryocystography. *Radiol. Clinics N. Am.* **10**:129 (1972).

6. Rogers, R. T.: Radiation Dose to the Skin in Diagnostic Radiography. *Br. J. Radiol.* **42:**511 (1969).

7. Chandler, A. C., Jr., and Wadsworth, J. A. C.: Conjunctivo-Dacryocystostomy: A Modified Conjunctivo-Dacryocystorhinostomy. *Trans. Am. Ophthalmol. Soc.* **71:**272 (1973).

8. Chandler, A. C., Jr., and Wadsworth, J. A. C.: Conjunctivodacryocystostomy. *Am. J. Ophthalmol.* **77:**830 (1974).

Intraocular Dynamic Function Studies in Nuclear Ophthalmology

Donald P. D'Amato, Ph.D.

Assistant Professor of Ophthalmology,
Division of Ophthalmology,
University of Connecticut Health Center,
Farmington, Connecticut

J. O'Rourke, M.D.

Professor and Chairman,
Department of Ophthalmology,
University of Connecticut Health Center,
Farmington, Connecticut

Charles Miller, M.D.

Clinical Associate of Theoretical
Physics,
Department of Ophthalmology,
University of Connecticut Health Center,
Farmington, Connecticut

J. Bronzino, M.D.

Clinical Consultant,
Biological Engineering,
University of Connecticut Health Center,
Farmington, Connecticut

When one desires to measure some function of the eye, generally one would like to make that measurement (or most any measurement for that matter) under equilibrium conditions; that is, under conditions in which the eye is disturbed as slightly as possible from its "normal" state. Some conventional measurements of eye functions (such as tonography) are made under nonequilibrium conditions. Nuclear tracer techniques, however, offer the possibility of making these elusive equilibrium measurements possible.

Tracer techniques are invasive only during a very short, initial period. Once the tracer is in the eye, its concentration is so low that it may usually be neglected biologically. Eye functions may then be monitored by means of an external noncontact probe. Typically, the eye function under study is rather slow, characterized by a few percent per minute tracer turnover rate. This slow rate necessitates a rather long time baseline for its accurate measurement. The clearance of a tracer from most any compartment displays an exponential behavior with time. Changes in the clearance rate are easily visualized when the data are displayed in semilog fashion. Therefore, it is imperative to logarithmically convert the counts obtained by the nuclear detection system prior to display. Once converted, the counts per time interval may be least squares fitted with a straight line and the clearance rate accurately measured.

EQUIPMENT AND TECHNIQUE

About 2 years ago, our research group realized that while the procedures of accurate counting over long baselines with subsequent logarithmic conversion and least squares fitting might be accomplished by conventional nuclear counting equipment and a suitable calculator, a small programmable computer would be ideal for the task. The computer might also semiautomate the previously manual procedures of data acquisition, recording, and plotting. Thus, the computer could control equipment and accumulate data and still have free time to perform real time computations of that data. Results of the computations, along with a semilog plot of the data, would be available during or immediately following the procedure that was performed on the eye. In the past 2 years, we have assembled such an automatic system.

The front end of the system is the gamma probe itself (Fig. 1). It was designed specifically for the measurement of the clearance of low energy gamma-emitting tracers from the eye. In order to minimize counting rate artifacts due to patient motion, the gamma detector must be suitably distant from the eye. In our case, we have chosen a distance of 4–6 in. Because the eye is not tolerant of high radiation dosage and the source-to-detector distance is rather large, the detector must be efficient. We have used a NaI (Tl) crystal of 5 in. diameter, coupled to a 5 in. phototube. The crystal is ¼ in. thick and has a .005 in. aluminum entrance window. It is quite efficient for gamma rays below 140 keV energy ($\sim$80% of incoming photons are recorded in the photopeak at 122 keV). The supporting structure is ⅝ in. stainless steel and also serves as shielding against stray radiation coming from regions other than the eye. (There is approximately 1% transmission through ⅝ in. steel for gamma radiation of 100 keV.)

The linear signals from the phototube are amplified, analyzed, and counted by standard NIM electronics. The NIM scaler is controlled and read by the computer. The computer is a PDP-8E manufactured by Digital Equipment Corporation, and the scaler is interfaced to the computer by an interface designed and constructed by our research

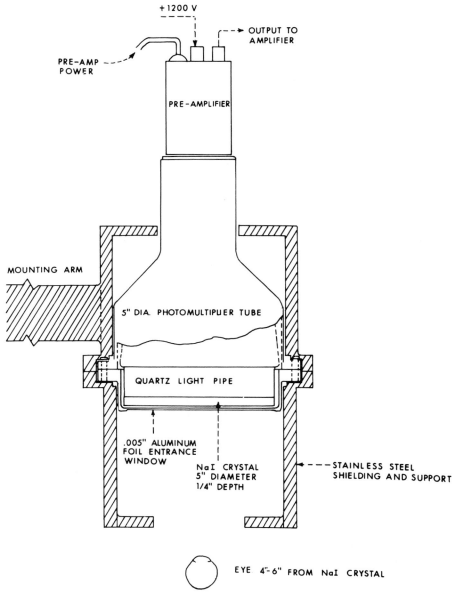

+1200 V

OUTPUT TO
AMPLIFIER

PRE-AMP
POWER

PRE-AMPLIFIER

MOUNTING ARM

5" DIA. PHOTOMULTIPLIER TUBE

QUARTZ LIGHT PIPE

.005" ALUMINUM
FOIL ENTRANCE
WINDOW

NaI CRYSTAL
5" DIAMETER
1/4" DEPTH

STAINLESS STEEL
SHIELDING AND SUPPORT

EYE 4"-6" FROM NaI CRYSTAL

Fig. 1.

group, utilizing two D.E.C. modules. The computer presently has 16K of core memory, which enables programs of moderate complexity to be run along with a large amount of memory devoted to data storage. A block diagram of our instrument system is shown in Fig. 2.

The piece of equipment that, to a very large extent, determines the usefulness of a minicomputer is the I/O terminal that is connected to it. We have utilized a Tektronix 4010 Interactive Graphics Terminal. With this device, we can output mixed graphics

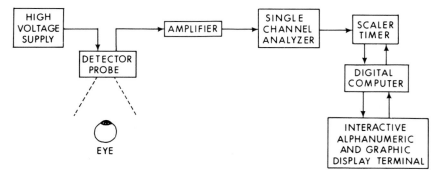

Fig. 2.

and alphanumerics at a very high speed: 9600 baud or about 1000 characters of alphanumerics per second. The display is of the persistence type so that the computer memory is not committed to refreshing the screen. A hard copy of the display may be obtained at any time by an accessory hard copy unit that produces 8½ × 11 in. paper copies of the display. One feature of the terminal that we have found exceptionally useful is a cross-hair cursor that allows the operator to interact with the computer to choose regions of interest on graphs for possible rescaling or fitting. This feature is comparable to the "light-pen" found on some computer terminals or gamma cameras.

In order for the data and the computer programs to be efficiently stored and recalled when needed, a mass storage device is desirable. We have used magnetic cassettes as the mass storage medium. Although somewhat slow, in a clinical environment, they have proven simple and convenient to use, especially by people untrained in computer techniques. With the amount of data presently generated per patient, we can store 50 to 100 patient records on a single cassette. Any one of these records may be recalled for analysis and examination within a few minutes.

When we first decided that computer automation was a way of greatly improving radioisotope clearance studies, we looked for a software or programming system that might be readily adaptable to our use. We originally felt that a D.E.C. Real Time BASIC might be appropriate, and actually, several of the earlier programs we developed were written in this BASIC. However, BASIC proved cumbersome in use because it had to be extensively modified by special overlays for each particular type of equipment we wished to control. Since then, we have been utilizing FORTRAN instead. FORTRAN has the capability of incorporating relocatable assembly language subroutines. A different assembly language routine was written for each device to be controlled and only called in when needed. Additionally, FORTRAN easily makes use of the full 16K of core memory, whereas BASIC would have to be specially modified to do so.

We now have considerable experience programming in FORTRAN and a compatible assembly language called SABR. We have written many main routines and subroutines. Routines have been written for real-time radioisotope clearance work, for storage and retrieval of data, and for the storage of studies done prior to the acquisition of the computer; also, several programs were written for automating and simplifying the procedure of tonography. To see the improvements that might be gained by computer control and analysis, we might take a look at some of the results of the various types of studies we have done.

Figure 3 is a semilog plot of the counts recorded every half-minute following intracameral injection of saline solution of ^{133}Xe in a patient study. The dashed line is a 5% per minute reference line. The counts in each half-minute are recorded as a cross with the initial counts set equal to 100%. For the first 23 minutes, the data closely follows the 5% per minute reference line. At about 23 minutes, Neo-Synephrine (10%) was administered topically to the eye. There was, at first, an artifact due to some patient motion, but then the clearance slope settled down. Least squares fitting was done on the clearance data from 0 to 22 minutes, and from 24.5 to 37 minutes. As may be seen, the fits show that the drug slowed the xenon clearance—from about 5.4% per minute to about 4.1% per minute.

Figure 4 is a patient tonogram plotted and analyzed by the eye physiometer. The computer has automatically scaled and timed the tonogram. The vertical scale is the usual 0 to 20 Schiötz scale, while on the horizontal is the time in minutes. At the end of 4 minutes, the computer program performs a least squares fitting of the data to a straight line and calculates the initial and final scale readings, the initial and final intraocular pressures and the coefficient of outflow ("C") in microliters per minute per millimeter of mercury.

Figure 5 is a demonstration of the sophistication of calculation that may be achieved by the present configuration of the physiometer with 16K of core memory. The graph is a plot of the clearance of xenon from a cat's eye. The upper set of data (the crosses) represent the counts recorded per minute expressed as a percent of initial count. There is an obvious bend in the clearance slope, perhaps indicating that clearance is from more

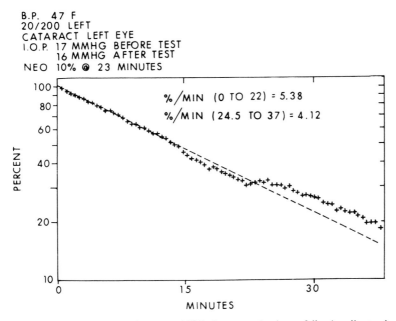

Fig. 3. Semilogarithmic graph of the clearance of ^{133}Xe from a patient's eye following direct microinjection. The dashed line is a reference slope of 5% per minute.

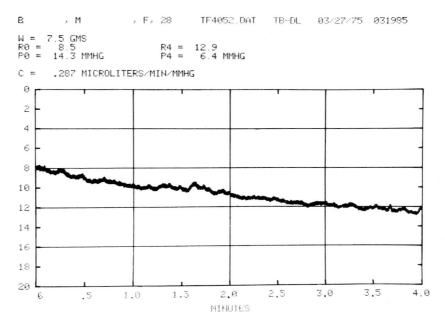

Fig. 4.   Patient tonogram; timed, plotted, and analyzed by computer.

CT153B.DAT   XE-PI   11/21/74   003594

PERCENT/MIN - 1 (58.0 TO 89.0) = 2.187 (+-) .018   CHI**2/DF =   1.37
PERCENT/MIN - 2 (.0 TO 31.0) = 7.172 (+-) .017   CHI**2/DF =   1.17

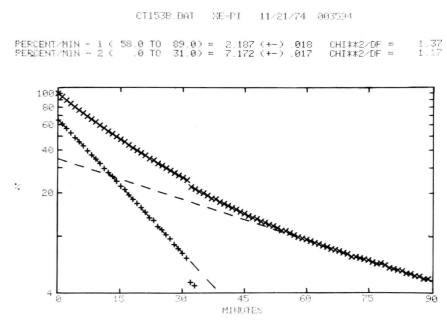

Fig. 5.   Semilog graph of ^{133}Xe clearance from feline eye with fitting and stripping. Dashed lines are fitted slopes.

than a single physiological compartment. A least squares fit was performed on this data from 58 to 89 minutes. One of the dashed lines is this calculated fit. This calculated fit was then subtracted from the data. The counts obtained by this subtraction were plotted and are seen as the plus signs. The subtracted data were then least squares fitted (from 0 to 31 minutes), and this fit is seen as the second dashed line. The corresponding clearance rates with associated standard errors and quality of fit (chi-squared per degree of freedom) parameters are displayed above the graph. The fact that the subtracted data is quite straight, as indicated both by eye and by the quality of fit, show that the xenon clearance may most probably be represented by a two compartment model.

CLINICAL RELATIONSHIP

The significance of dynamic function studies lies in the area of clinical eye physiology. It is no secret that ophthalmology suffers from a shortage of in vivo, quantitative information about the physiological aspects of its major diseases. Because of this, it seems to me that dynamic function studies represent a prime area for collaboration between ophthalmology and nuclear medicine.

In developing useful, dynamic function studies for the eye, one must deal with certain obstacles. These have been detailed elsewhere[1] but may be outlined as follows.

First, the limbus—the anterior chamber is the only dynamic physiological compartment located on the body surface. It is also one of the few whose dynamics have not been measured in patients by the essential method of tracer kinetics analysis. The drawback here has been our inability to achieve selective localization and mixing of tracers within this compartment following systemic administration.

Second, mathematics—it is generally known that physicians have not been inclined to utilize mathematics in the solution of clinical problems, and that mathematicians have been equally reluctant to express clinical concepts in a readable, narrative form.

Third, disparate methodology in eye physiology. Progress in the clinical physiology of any organ or system requires the opportunity to utilize similar methods of procedure and data presentation in basic and clinical laboratories.

Fourth, a time conflict in eye physiology. Disparate methods are used because dynamic functions of the eye exhibit slow rates of change. Long-term continuous measurements are needed if such functions are to be accurately measured. Unfortunately, the eye does not tolerate prolonged physical contact, including the cannulations on which many basic studies in eye physiology have depended.

There are other technological problems that may affect the effort to relate ophthalmology to nuclear medicine, but these four are most fundamental.

Delta entry of tracer by limbal micropuncture (Fig. 6) achieves selective localization and mixing. It also simplifies the mathematical approach to measurements of dynamic clearance. It does so by enabling one to reduce the assumptions and calculations to relatively simple first- or second-order equations to be computed by the instrumentation. Systemic or transcorneal administration (iontophoresis) presents a spectrum of rates of tracer entry in a drawn out process that greatly complicates the mathematical calculation of tracer washout.

Two concepts most vital to clinical physiology everywhere (Fig. 7) are expotential expressions of time-dependent rate changes from calculus and the computation of accuracy based on laws of statistics and probability. Our reluctance to apply them to the

DELTA ENTRY VS MATH

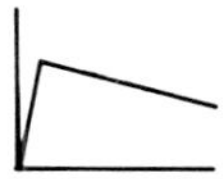

RAPID ENTRY AND RAPID MIXING IN COMPARTMENT.

CONFINE CHANGE TO REGION COMPARTMENT OUTLET.

REDUCE ASSUMPTIONS: ALLOW USE FIRST ORDER EQUATIONS.

PERMIT USE DIGITAL DATA AND COMPUTER AIDS.

Fig. 6.

management of clinical problems is rapidly yielding to the enticements of computer science and the presence of physical scientists in our clinical laboratories.

The main point about a time conflict mentioned earlier (Fig. 8) is that it has seriously limited the *amount* of information available from each eye patient studied. Anatomical, structural, and qualitative information, on the other hand, may be gathered in great quantities via direct observations and photography. As a result, anatomical diagnosis most often predominates in the management of eye diseases caused primarily by physiological changes. Accuracy in clinical diagnosis, largely depends on the *amount* of quantitative information available. This statistical concept of standard deviation applies to eye disease management. It simply indicates that the needed amounts of physiological information must be recovered by prolonging the period of measurement (using nuclear methods) while minimizing the period of physical eye contact (by brief, initial microinjection).

Regarding microinjection, the assets of a lancet-pointed 30-gauge needle for easy piercing of the limbus have been described in a recent publication.[1] Conventional, single-bevel needles and surgical methods for paracentesis are inadequate for these studies because a self-sealing low resistance micropuncture is not achieved. When mounted on a gas-tight 50 μl chromatography syringe, we find this 30-gauge point very useful.

Concerning dynamic studies and their interpretation, consider the situation in aqueous bulk flow. In Figs. 9 and 10, the washout of [125]Iodine labeled human serum albumin from the feline anterior chamber is depicted. Similar studies have been done in patients with glaucoma.[1] The clearance proceeds as a monoexponential slope once pressure has recovered after microinjection (20 μl, 5 μCi). Topical administration of pilocarpine accelerates and water loading slows the clearance. In similar studies of xenon

MATH VS CLINICAL DYNAMIC FUNCTIONS

RATE & TIME – DEPENDENCE ARE DIFF. CAL. CONCEPTS.

ACCURACY AS FUNCTION OF DATA AMOUNT IS STAT. CONCEPT.

PHYSICIANS RELUCTANT TO APPLY MATH. TO CLIN. PROBLEMS.

NUCLEAR COUNTING & COMPUTER AID SPEED MATH. APPLICATIONS.

Fig. 7.

TIME VS ACCURACY

GRADUAL RATES REQUIRE LONG, CONTINUOUS MEASUREMENT.

EYE TOLERANCE LIMITS PERIOD OF PHYSICAL CONTACT.

INFO. SHORTAGE EXISTS IN RE DYNAMIC ASPECTS DISEASE.

ACCURACY IN MATH AND IN DX DEPENDS UPON <u>AMT.</u> OF INFO.

INFINITELY HIGH AMTS. GIVE INFINITELY HIGH ACCURACY.

Fig. 8.

CAT. NO. 4179   10/6/73 125 IALB A.C. WASHOUT
PILO 4% @ 23 MIN.
KETAMINE, ANES.

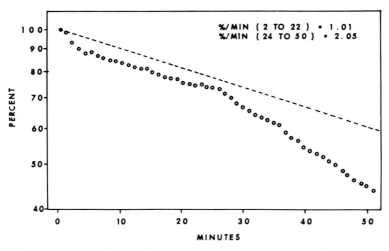

Fig. 9. ^{125}I-HSA clearance from feline eye. Pilocarpine —4% drops administered at 23 minutes.

CAT. NO. 10226 125 IALB. A.C. WASHOUT 1/4/74
I.V. DEXTROSE 5% 60 CC @ 90 MIN.
URETHANE, ANES.

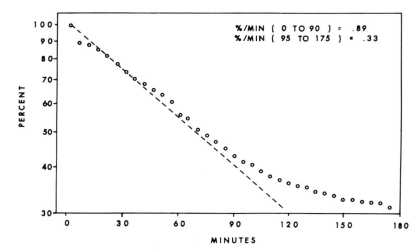

Fig. 10. ^{125}I-HSA clearance from feline eye; 60 cc of 5% dextrose injected intravenously at 90 minutes to simulate a water provocative test.

clearance the capillary flow in the anterior segment is measured and computer analyzed (Fig. 3).

SUMMARY

Clinical ophthalmology is deficient in clinical knowledge of the invisible intraocular dynamic functions. These usually determine the course and outcome of its major diseases. In seeking to study them, a sensible collaboration with the rapidly growing specialties of nuclear medicine and medical physics should be arranged. Key requirements include selective localization and mixing of tracers in the anterior chamber by brief microinjection, simplification of computations by attention to the simplification of instrumental design, and the use of similar methods for measurement of dynamic function in basic and clinical laboratories. These seem to be the present needs of clinical eye physiology.

REFERENCE

1. O'Rourke, J.: Measurements of Capillary Function in Eye Diseases. *Trans. Am. Ophthalmol. Soc.* **72**:606–649 (1974).

The Orbit and Adnexae

STATIC STUDIES

Physiological Basis
of Exophthalmos

James C. Sisson, M.D.
Professor of Internal Medicine,
Section of Nuclear Medicine,
University of Michigan Medical Center,
Ann Arbor, Michigan

To describe the physiological basis for thyroid exophthalmos, the ophthalmopathy of Graves' disease, is a pretentious undertaking. Although Robert Graves described the disorder 140 years ago, the many facets and interrelationships that make up Graves' disease have only begun to unravel. Recent investigations appear to have opened some secrets and have excited the imaginations of endocrinologists and ophthalmologists alike.

DEFINITIONS

Important as background information is the clinical nature of Graves' disease. The disorder is recognized by the clinical manifestations (Table 1) which are multiple, but frequently not all are present in an afflicted individual. Worthy of note is that the extrathyroidal manifestations, including Graves' eye disease, arise independently of the thyroidal changes. Thus the ophthalmopathy, dermopathy, and acropachy, although uniquely related to Graves' disease, are not caused by increases in circulating thyroid hormones.

The ophthalmopathy has occurred before, after, and simultaneously with hyperthyroidism.[1] About 4 to 5% of patients develop Graves' eye disease but never experience hyperthyroidism. Conversely, 30 to 40% of patients suffer from the effects of hypersecretion of thyroid hormones but are free of ocular abnormality.

Graves' ophthalmopathy is recognized by the individual and collective features in the orbital and periorbital areas. The American Thyroid Association adopted the classification for eye changes seen in Table 2.[2] Categorization by this scheme (which includes subclasses not shown in Table 2) benefits the care of patients in two ways. First, a particular clinical problem is clarified. Since each patient generally develops only a few of the ocular features, a given individual's affliction and disability are precisely perceived when so classified, goals not achieved when the generic term "exophthalmos" is used. Second, the separate ocular features frequently exhibit different natural histories.[3] For example, soft tissue swelling frequently diminishes as the activity of the disease process disappears, but proptosis and extraocular muscle inbalance generally improve little, if at all. Plans for, and evaluations of, therapies directed at Graves' ophthalmopathy must take into account the identifiable ophthalmologic changes and their probable course if the physician does not intervene.

EVALUATIONS OF PHYSIOLOGICAL AND PATHOLOGICAL HORMONAL RELATIONSHIPS

In the process of seeking laboratory aids for diagnosis of Graves' disease, much has been learned about the relationship of the thyroid gland to the pituitary gland and the

TABLE 1.   CLINICAL EXPRESSIONS OF GRAVES' DISEASE

A. Thyroidal
    1.   Diffuse hyperplasia (goiter)
    2.   Hypersecretion of thyroid hormones and consequent hyperthyroidism
B. Extrathyroidal
    1.   Ophthalmopathy (exophthalmos)
    2.   Dermopathy (pretibial myxedema)
    3.   Acropachy (clubbing of digits and/or periosteal proliferation)

TABLE 2. CLASSIFICATION OF FEATURES OF GRAVES'
OPHTHALMOPATHY[a]

Class Number
0. No signs or symptoms
1. Only signs, no symptoms (minor proptosis and/or lid retraction)
2. Soft tissue swelling (symptoms and signs)
3. Proptosis (more marked than in Class 2)
4. Extraocular muscle involvement
5. Corneal involvement (keratitis)
6. Sight loss (optic nerve changes)

[a] Adopted by the American Thyroid Association[2].

hypothalamus. Generally, there is little problem in arriving at the correct diagnosis when hyperthyroidism has been identified at some time in a patient's course of disease. However, when ocular changes appear without hyperthyroidism, and especially if the eye manifestations are atypical (e.g., the disease may begin in one eye), some help to confirm clinical suspicions is welcome. It is, of course, mandatory to exclude processes in the orbit other than Graves' disease.

Although the presence of dermopathy or of long-acting thyroid stimulator (LATS) in the serum identify the disorder, these components of Graves' disease occur infrequently and are usually absent in the patient who presents the diagnostic problem.

Many patients who are euthyroid but suffer from ophthalmopathy have developed functional changes in the thyroid gland which are characteristic of Graves' disease but require special tests for detection. *Apparent autonomy of thyroid function (unsuppressible when thyroid hormones are administered, even in large doses) is frequently observed in patients with severe and active Graves' eye disease.*[4]

The homeostasis of the pituitary-thyroid relationship (Fig. 1) can now be evaluated by recording serum thyrotropin (TSH) responses to injections of a modulator from the hypothalamus, thyrotropin-releasing hormone (TRH). Serial values of TSH are reproducible and peak at 30 minutes after an intravenous injection of TRH. Small increases in the concentrations of circulating thyroid hormones, thyroxine (T4) and triiodothyronine (T3), suppress the TSH responses;[5] conversely, small decreases in the quantities of secreted thyroid hormones result in exaggerated rises in TSH after the injection of TRH.[6] These abnormal TSH patterns are very sensitive indices of altered thyroid function and may be observed in the absence of other evidence of dysfunction (e.g., the patient may appear clinically euthyroid.) *In patients who develop Graves'*

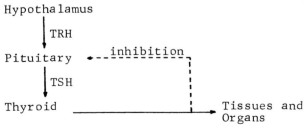

Fig. 1.   The Pituitary thyroid relationship.

ophthalmopathy, without hyperthyroidism, frequently the TSH responses to TRH are suppressed or exaggerated, indicating minor degrees of thyroid functional abnormalities in these subjects.[7, 8] The diagnostic value of this type of laboratory evaluation is obvious, but, for this discussion, it is especially important to note that the pituitary responses are what one would predict from the known physiological relationships between thyroid and pituitary glands. Therefore, it appears that the pituitary, and, by extrapolation, also the hypothalamus, are not primarily at fault in Graves' disease; the aberrations in thyroid function arise autonomously or via some paraendocrine stimulation.

ALTERED IMMUNE SYSTEM IN GRAVES' DISEASE

Some clues to the basic nature of Graves' disease are found in the histologic changes of the affected tissues. In the orbit, three major microscopic features are visible[9]: (*1*) infiltrations of lymphocytes; (*2*) increased quantities of ground substance, identified as hydrophilic glycosaminoglycans (GAG), particularly hyaluronic acid; and (*3*) fibrosis, which ultimately supervenes. Aggregations of lymphocytes are commonly encountered also in the thyroid glands of patients with Graves' disease. The infiltrations of tissues by lymphocytes, the lymphocytosis in the blood,[10] and the enlarged thymus glands[11] found in afflicted individuals point to a disturbance in the immune system. Further, the widespread manifestations of Graves' disease suggest that circulating factors, which might include lymphocytes and immune globulin, play a role in pathogenesis. Although separation of immune responses into those related to antibody formation by B lymphocytes (derived from the bone marrow) and those arising from cell-mediated changes by T lymphocytes (derived from the thymus gland) is an oversimplification of a complex system, it is convenient to record the abnormalities observed in patients with Graves' disease by this scheme.

Antibody (Immune Globulin) Formation

Table 3 lists the types of antibodies that have been commonly detected in patients with Graves' disease. The production of antithyroid antibodies is somewhat more characteristic of Hashimoto's disease; however, it has been proposed that Graves' disease and Hashimoto's thyroiditis are at opposite ends of a clinical-histologic spectrum of a single autoimmune disorder.[12]

LATS clearly stimulates thyroid function, but it is now thought that this immune globulin is not pathogenic for most, if any, patients since there is but weak correlation

TABLE 3.   ALTERATIONS IN B (BONE MARROW-DERIVED) LYMPHOCYTE
FUNCTION IN GRAVES' DISEASE

1. Antibodies produced against components of thyroid tissue:
    a.   Thyroglobulin
    b.   Microsomal fraction
2. Long-acting thyroid stimulator (LATS): an immune globulin found only in patients with Graves' disease but for which no defined antigen has been found.
3. LATS protector: another immune globulin found only in patients with Graves' disease and for which the antigen is not known.

TABLE 4.   ALTERATIONS IN T (THYMUS-DERIVED) LYMPHOCYTE
           FUNCTION IN GRAVES' DISEASE

1. From patients with active disease, lymphocytes produce migration inhibition factor opon ex-
    posure to:
    a. Crude thyroid tissue antigen
    b. Extraocular muscle antigen[16]
2. From patients with active disease, the numbers and activity of T lymphocytes are increased[17]
3. Plaque formation through the interaction of T and B lymphocytes (indicating sensitized and
    active T lymphocytes) is abnormally increased by cells from:
    a. Patients with active disease
    b. Patients with inactive disease (but responses are less than in a)
    c. Many relatives of patients with Graves' disease[18]

between the presence of LATS and the clinical and hormonal activities of Graves'
disease.[13] LATS-protector is a more recently discovered immune globulin, which, in addition to protecting LATS from neutralization by thyroid tissue, stimulates thyroid function itself.[14] Although LATS-protector could be an important mediator of thyroid functional abnormalities, it almost certainly plays no role in Graves' ophthalmopathy.[15]

Cell-mediated Immune Activity

One of the most sensitive indicators of cell-mediated immune activity has been the in
vitro production of migration inhibition factor (MIF) by T lymphocytes. MIF is
released by T cells previously sensitized to a particular antigen when this antigen is included in the incubation medium. The presence and quantity of MIF are measured by
recording the inhibition of migration of mixed leukocytes associated with the
lymphocytes in culture. Lymphocytes from patients with Graves' disease produce MIF
upon exposure to a crude thyroid antigen (Fig. 2).[16] In this system, significant MIF was
invariably released by lymphocytes of patients who exhibited clinical hyperthyroidism,
but the results were more varied for cells obtained from individuals who manifested
ophthalmopathy without hyperthyroidism.

Conversely, upon exposure to retroorbital muscle antigen, lymphocytes from subjects
suffering ocular disease consistently produced MIF, but those from patients with only
hyperthyroidism were less predictable in this assay (Fig. 3). One interpretation of these
results is that at least two antigens, one from thyroid and another from orbital muscle,
are involved in the cell-mediated immune responses in Graves' disease.

The investigators who have developed the above data have also reported that the
absolute number (per milliliter of blood) of circulating T lymphocytes and the functional
activity of these cells (when inhibited by antithymocyte globulin) are significantly
increased above normal values in patients with Graves' disease.[17] Further, the degree of
laboratory abnormality agreed with clinical activity of the disorder.

Another approach to measuring cell-mediated responses was reported by the same
investigators at a recent meeting.[18] Cooperation between B and T lymphocytes was
assessed by noting that immunologically active (from recent exposure to antigen to
which they are sensitized) T cells induce, in culture, the surrounding B cells to produce
an IgM globulin. This, in turn, lyses sheep erythrocytes, which are added to the assay

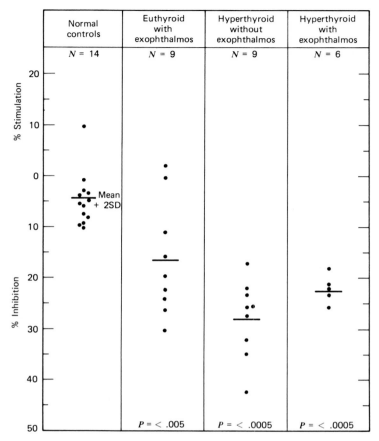

Fig. 2. Percent inhibition of leukocyte migration to thyroid antigen in untreated Graves' disease. (Reproduced from reference 16 with permission.)

system. The lysed erythrocytes appear as plaques which are counted and related to the volume of blood from which the lymphocytes were separated. The results correlated with the presence and the clinical activity, both in the thyroid and in the orbit, of Graves' disease. Moreover, many relatives of patients with Graves' disease had lymphocytes which produced an abnormal number of plaques by this technique. Although a common environmental factor cannot be excluded as a factor, the data lend support to the concept of a genetic predisposition for Graves' disease via the immune system.

If the pathogenesis of Graves' disease derives from autoimmunity, the question of how the immunologic processes elicit the cellular and functional changes of the involved tissues requires an answer. It is possible that T and B lymphocytes work together in the thyroid, eventually producing a LATS-protector and LATS which, singly or together, bring about an "autonomous" hyperthyroidism. In the orbit, the synthesis of large quantities of GAG may result from direct interaction of lymphocytes and connective tissue cells. In cultures of fibroblasts derived from human orbital connective tissue, the addition of lymphocytes evoked increased synthesis of GAG by the former.[19] This

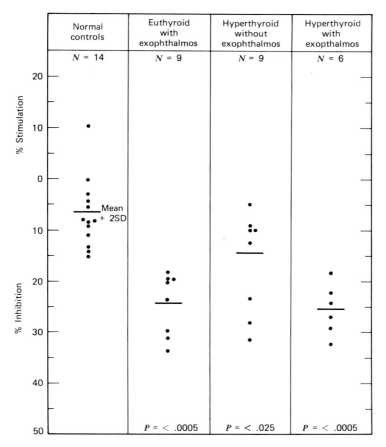

Fig. 3. Percent inhibition of leukocyte migration to retroorbital muscle antigen in untreated Graves' disease. (Reproduced from reference 16 with permission.)

cellular interaction is not dependent upon immunologically sensitized lymphocytes, since cells from normal subjects produced almost the same results. However, the immune disturbance may attract the lymphocytes to the orbital tissues, which then nonspecifically react to the infiltration by an outpouring of hydrophilic GAG.

IMPLICATIONS OF THE DATA

The available information is sufficient to indict but not yet convict an altered immune system for the crime of Graves' disease. Probably individuals who develop Graves' disease are genetically predisposed to this malady. A population study led to the conclusion that such an inherited susceptibility indeed exists.[20]

Efficacy has not been clearly established for any of the proposed therapies for Graves' eye disease. However, if one assumes that the several nonsurgical treatments provide benefit to at least some patients, then it is interesting to note that the four major approaches to the eye problem, now in use, act against the immune system. Large doses of corticosteroids[21] and x-irradiation[22, 23] have been employed for many years to help reverse the serious ocular changes of Graves' disease. Although these treatment modalities were not originally adopted to alter autoimmunity, their effects on immune responses are clearly established. Azathiaprine, an agent commonly employed to impair immune reactions, has more recently been advocated as prophylaxis against the development of Graves' ophthalmopathy in patients who exhibit hyperthyroidism.[24] Finally, to remove all thyroid cells, large doses of ^{131}I have been administered to patients who manifest advanced orbital changes.[25] This approach is based on the premise that lymphocytes of individuals with Graves' disease have been sensitized by a thyroidal antigen and the immune responses also involve a cross-reacting orbital antigen; elimination of the original inciting antigen should then break the cycle of autoimmune disease.

Future investigations will further untangle the enigma of Graves' disease. With the understanding gained through these endeavors, not only can better therapies be logically planned but prevention may also be possible.

REFERENCES

1. Bartels, E. C., and Irie, M.: In Pitt-Rivers, R., Ed., *Advances in Thyroid Research*. New York. Pergamon, 1961, p. 163.
2. Werner, S. C.: Classification of the Eye Changes of Graves' Disease. *J. Clin. Endocrinol. Metab.* **29**:982–984 (1969).
3. Riise, R.: Long-term Prognosis in Malignant Exophthalmos. *Acta Ophthalmol.* **48**:634–643 (1970).
4. Ivy, H. K.: Medical Approach to Ophthalmopathy of Graves' Disease. *Mayo Clin. Proc.* **47**:980–985 (1972).
5. Snyder, P. J., and Utiger, R. D.: Inhibition of Thyrotropin Response to Thyrotropin-releasing Hormone by Small Quantities of Thyroid Hormones. *J. Clin. Invest.* **51**:2077–2084 (1972).
6. Vagenakis, A. G., Rapoport, B., Azizi, F. et al: Hyperresponse to Thyrotropin-releasing Hormone Accompanying Small Decreases in Serum Thyroid Hormone Concentrations. *J. Clin. Invest.* **54**:913–918 (1974).
7. Chopra, I., Chopra, U., and Orgiazzi, J.: Abnormalities of Hypothalamo-Hypophyseal-Thyroid Axis in Patients with Graves' Ophthalmopathy. *J. Clin. Endocrinol. Metab.* **37**:955–966 (1973).
8. Clifton-Bligh, P., Silverstein, G. E., and Burke, G.: Unresponsiveness to Thyrotropin-releasing Hormone (TRH) in Treated Graves' Hyperthyroidism and in Euthyroid Graves' Disease. *J. Clin. Endocrinol. Metab.* **38**:531–537 (1974).
9. Riley, F. C.: Orbital Pathology in Graves' Disease. *Mayo Clin. Proc.* **47**:975–979 (1972).
10. Wallerstein, R. O., and Cassell, W. B.: In Werner, S. C., and Ingbar, S. H., Eds., *The Thyroid*, 3rd ed. Harper and Row, New York, 1971, p. 640.
11. Michie, W., Beck, J. S., and Mahaffey, R. G.: Quantitative Radiological and Histological Studies of the Thymus in Thyroid Disease. *Lancet* **1**:691–695 (1967).
12. Hall, R., Doniach, D., Kirkham, K. et al: Ophthalmic Graves' Disease. *Lancet* **1**:375–378 (1970).
13. Chopra, I. J., Solomon, D. E., Johnson, D. E. et al: Thyroid Gland in Graves' Disease: Victim or Culprit? *Metabolism* **19**:760–772 (1970).
14. Adams, D. D., Fastier, F. N., Howie, J. B. et al: Stimulation of the Human Thyroid by Infusions of Plasma Containing LATS Protector. *J. Clin. Endocrinol. Metab.* **39**:826–832 (1974).
15. Adams, D. D., Kennedy, T. H., and Stewart, R. D. H.: Correlation Between Long-acting Thyroid Stimulator Protector Level and Thyroid [131]I Uptake in Thyrotoxicosis. *Br. Med. J.* **2**:199–201 (1974).
16. Munro, R. E., Lamki, L., Row, V. V. et al: Cell-mediated Immunity in the Exophthalmos of Graves' Disease as Demonstrated by the Migration Inhibition Factor (MIF) Test. *J. Clin. Endocrinol. Metab.* **37**:286–292 (1973).
17. Farid, N. R., Munro, R., Row, V. V. et al: Rosette Inhibition Test for the Demonstration of Thymus-dependent Lymphocyte Sensitization in Graves' Disease and Hashimoto's Thyroiditis. *N. Engl. J. Med.* **289**:111–1117 (1973).

18.   Farid, N. R., Von Westarp, C., Row, V. V. et al: Interaction Between Thymus-dependent (T) and Bursa-equivalent (B) Lymphocytes in Human Thyroid Disease Demonstrated by Direct Plaque Formation. Presented at the Annual American Thyroid Association Meeting in St. Louis, Sept. 20, 1974.

19.   Sisson, J. C.: Stimulation of Glucose Utilization and Glycosaminoglycans Production by Fibroblasts Derived from Retrobulbar Tissue. *Exp. Eye Res.* **2**:285–292 (1971).

20.   Volpe, R., Edmonds, M., Lamki, L. et al: The Pathogenesis of Graves' Disease: A Disorder of Delayed Hypersensitivity? *Mayo Clin. Proc.* **47**:824–834 (1972).

21.   Werner, S. C.: Prednisone in Emergency Treatment of Malignant Exophthalmos. *Lancet* **1**:1004–1007 (1966).

22.   Donaldson, S. S., Bagshaw, M. A., and Kriss, J. P.: Supervoltage Orbital Radiotherapy for Graves' Ophthalmopathy. *J. Clin. Endocrinol. Metab.* **37**:276–285 (1973).

23.   Ravin, J. G., Sisson, J. C., and Knapp, W. T.: Orbital Radiation for the Ocular Changes of Graves' Disease. *Am. J. Ophthalmol.* **79**:285–288 (1975).

24.   Winand, R., and Mahiew, P.: Prevention of Malignant Exophthalmos after Treatment of Thyrotoxicosis. *Lancet* **1**:1196 (1973).

25.   Blum, A. S., Greenspan, F. S., and Powell, M. R.: High Dose Radioactive Therapy for Infiltrative Ophthalmopathy of Graves' Disease. Presented at the Annual Meeting of American Thyroid Association in St. Louis, Sept. 20, 1974.

GENERAL READING

Brown, J., Chopra, I. J., Cornell, J. S. et al: Thyroid Physiology in Health and Disease. *Ann. Intern. Med.* **81**:68–81 (1974).

Kriss, J. P.: Graves' Ophthalmopathy: Etiology and Treatment. *Hosp. Practice* **10**:125–134 (March 1975).

Radioisotopes in Orbital Disease

Joseph C. Flanagan, M.D.
Senior Assistant Surgeon,
Oculoplastic Service,
Wills Eye Hospital;
Clinical Associate Professor,
Thomas Jefferson University,
Philadelphia, Pennsylvania

Orbital lesions are most commonly manifested by protrusion of the eye, clinically called exophthalmos or proptosis. Whether or not a given lesion produces exophthalmos and if so to what degree depends on (1) the size of the lesion, (2) its character, (3) its position in the orbit, and (4) its effect on the extraocular muscles. There are more than 50 different lesions listed in the English literature that may cause proptosis.[1] The 20 most common causes of unilateral exophthalmos and their relative frequency have been tabulated by Reese and are shown in Table 1.[2] An all-inclusive classification of orbital conditions does not exist; however, they may be grouped into four main types as proposed by Henderson[3]: (1) orbital neoplasms and cyst, (2) endocrine exophthalmos, (3) inflammatory disorders (pseudotumor), and (4) vascular malformations (fistulas, varices, and aneurysms). This grouping does not include pseudoproptosis caused by (1) asymmetry of the bony orbit; (2) unilateral high myopia; (3) early mild hyperthyroidism which produces a unilateral retraction of the upper lid; (4) a relaxation of one or more of the rectus muscles resulting from either a paralysis or from a previous operation, during which one or more of the extraocular muscles was unduly recessed; and (5) a unilateral hydrophthalmos or buphthalmos secondary to congenital glaucoma.[2]

The cause of a unilateral proptosis may be extremely difficult to diagnose. To make a diagnosis, it is extremely important to have a complete history and an ocular examination, including visual acuity, visual fields, evaluation of extraocular motility,

TABLE 1. A SERIES OF 230 CONSECUTIVE CASES OF UNILATERAL EXPANDING LESIONS OF THE ORBIT STUDIED CAREFULLY

	Diagnosis	Incidence (percent)
1.	Thyroid ophthalmopathy	16
2.	Hemangiomas	12
3.	Malignant-lymphomas	10
4.	Chronic granulomas (pseudotumors)	8
5.	Lacrimal gland epithelial tumors	7
6.	Meningiomas	5
7.	Lymphangiomas	4
8.	Gliomas of the optic nerve	3
9.	Metastatic malignant tumors	3
10.	Peripheral nerve tumors	3
11.	Dermoid cysts	3
12.	Mucoceles	3
13.	Soft-part sarcomas (rhabdomyosarcoma, granular-cell myoblastoma, etc.)	3
14.	Aneurysms	2
15.	Angiosarcomas	2
16.	Osteomas	1
17.	Histiocytomas	1
18.	Sarcoids	1
19.	Others (one case each of: fibrous dysplasia, encephalocele, tuberculosis, myxoma, dacryoadenitis and posterior scleritis)	0.5 each
20.	Exophthalmos of unknown cause	10

ophthalmoscopic examination, tonometry, orbitonometry, auscultation of the orbit, and a systematic survey. Special examinations are also necessary, including skull and orbital x-rays, tomography, angiography, venography, orbitography, ultrasonography, thermography, and radioisotope scanning. The use of radioisotopes has proved very helpful in the diagnosis of orbital disorders.

Technetium scans have been most helpful in differentiating endocrine exophthalmos and benign cystic lesions from orbital tumors. Exact localization within the orbit is sometimes possible. Serial scans are helpful in assessing the growth of a tumor and in detecting persistence or recurrence after treatment.

The following considerations are important to the proper interpretation of an orbital scan.

1. An increased area of activity either unilaterally or bilaterally.
2. A pattern of diffuse or local asymmetry in isotope uptake.
3. Focal or diffuse isotope activity within the questionable area.
4. An orbital roentgenogram for comparison and topographic orientation.

The work-up of a patient with unilateral exophthalmos must include a T_3, T_4, and a radioactive iodine uptake suppression test in order to exclude endocrine involvement.[4] The scan pattern may be normal or abnormal in endocrine ophthalmopathy. In the case of orbital neoplasms, a focal collection of isotope activity may be seen in the tumor area. This focal concentration of activity would tend to differentiate the lesion from a diffuse activity pattern more characteristic of inflammatory lesions and vascular abnormalities. Vascular abnormalities may sometimes be differentiated by dynamic flow studies in which the blood-pool or vascular defect may be more clearly outlined.

The combined use of ^{197}Hg and technetium pertechnetate has been reported by Grove and Kotner[5] as an adjunct in the differential diagnosis of orbital pathology. The combined use of the separate radionuclides was more often associated with neoplasms (benign and malignant). Rhabdomyosarcomas were strongly positive with pertechnetate but negative or weakly positive with ^{197}Hg-chlormerodrin. In patients with orbital myositis secondary to endocrine ophthalmopathy, the pertechnetate scans showed areas of increased activity surrounding the inflamed extraocular muscles (ring pattern). Increased activity in the pertechnetate scan was also associated with vascular and inflammatory lesions. Whether or not such precise differentiation of lesions can always be expected by using combined isotope techniques is not known. Table 2 shows the findings on orbital scanning using ^{99m}technetium pertechnetate in 25 patients who presented with a unilateral exophthalmos. The distribution of cases cannot be considered as a representative sampling of a population of unilateral exophthalmos because these patients were first evaluated by an ophthalmologist as the primary physician. Those patients in whom the presence of a tumor was detected by conventional testing were less likely to have a radioisotope scan study than those in whom the cause of the exophthalmos was obscure.

Putterman[4] has suggested a rather compact routine for the evaluation of orbital tumors. Twelve days prior to admission to the hospital a 6-hour radioactive iodine uptake test is done on an outpatient basis. During the next 12 days, Cytomel (25 μg) three times daily is taken by the patient. On the twelfth day the patient is admitted to the hospital and a 6-hour radioactive iodine suppression test is performed. A complete eye exam, including visual fields, ophthalmodynamometry, exophthalmometer readings, and

TABLE 2

| | Patient | | | |
	Age	Sex	Diagnosis	Scan Result
1.	47	F	Endocrine ophthalmopathy	+
2.	53	F	Endocrine ophthalmopathy	−
3.	58	F	Endocrine ophthalmopathy	−
4.	28	F	Endocrine ophthalmopathy	−
5.	47	F	Endocrine ophthalmopathy	−
6.	46	M	Endocrine ophthalmopathy	−
7.	56	F	Endocrine ophthalmopathy	+
8.	54	M	Endocrine ophthalmopathy	−
9.	65	F	Inflammatory pseudotumor	+
10.	59	M	Inflammatory pseudotumor	+
11.	45	M	Dacryoadenitis	+
12.	17	M	Orbital cellulitis	+
13.	36	M	Inflammatory pseudotumors	+
14.	58	F	Inflammatory pseudotumors	+
16.	65	F	Metastatic breast carcinoma	−
17.	80	M	Malignant melanoma choroid with extra ocular extension	−
18.	22	M	Cystic lesion left orbit	−
19.	67	M	Benign mixed tumor lacrimal gland	+
20.	48	M	Dermoid cyst	−
21.	69	M	Meningioma left orbit	+
22.	45	F	Hemangioma left orbit	+
23.	40	F	Neurolemmoma	+
24.	59	M	Metastatic malignant melanoma	+
25.	67	M	Malignant lymphoma	−

auscultation of the orbit, is performed. A complete physical examination is performed including a pelvic and proctoscopic examination as indicated. Orbital scans are performed along with dynamic studies with ^{99m}technetium pertechnetate.

On the second day of hospitalization, multiple x-rays of the patient's optic foramina, sinuses and orbital tomograms are performed. Venography, orbitography and carotid arteriography are done if indicated. On the third day, ultrasonography of the orbit is performed, and the results of all the tests are evaluated. In this manner, a complete survey for suspected orbital pathology can be undertaken in a logical fashion.

TECHNIQUE

It has been customary in brain scanning to obtain anterior views by keeping the cantho-meatal line perpendicular to the detector. The use of this method obliterates activity normally present in the nasopharynx, paranasal sinuses, and parotid gland. As a result, the orbits and anterior part of the middle cranial fossa are not visible.

A number of authors[6, 7, 8] have delineated the basic method for obtaining the best information in orbital scan techniques. The technique involves the use of *en face* method

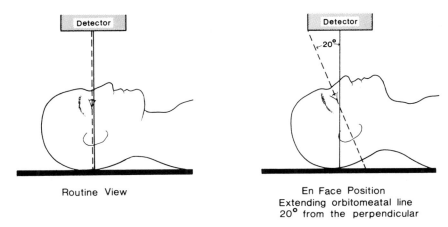

Fig. 1. Radionuclide scanning of the orbital areas utilizing the *en face* position (right) in contrast to the routine view (left). (Courtesy of E. B. Wilson, R. C. Briggs, *Radiology* 92:3 576–580, March 1969. Copyright 1969 The Radiological Society of North America Inc.)

of scanning similar to the radiographic technique used in the classic Waters view of the orbits, except that the patient is examined in the supine rather than the prone position. The cantho-meatal line is placed 15°–20° cephalad to the detector element thus rendering both orbits visible to the scan (Fig. 1). The scans are performed 1 hour after the intravenous administration of 10 mCi of technetium pertechnetate. Figure 2b shows the normal one-quarter axial anterior scan compared to the normal *en face* anterior scan (Fig. 2a) in schematic representation. It should be noted that in the *en face* scan, high activity areas are seen in the mouth, pharynx, nasal turbinate, mucous membranes, temporal muscles, and parotid glands. The cerebral hemispheres show less activity than the surrounding structures. Radiating outward from the middle activity is the area of the

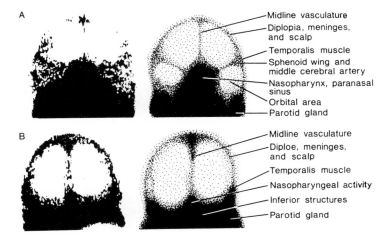

Fig. 2.   (*A*) Simulated scan view of orbital areas in *en face* position. (*B*) Simulated view of normal anterior brain scan. Note absence of orbital areas and sphenoid wing. (Courtesy of E. B. Wilson, R. C. Briggs, *Radiology* 92:3 576–580 March 1969. Copyright 1969 The Radiological Society of North American Inc.)

sphenoid wing and cerebral vessels. Inferior to this is the orbital area. Anterior middle fossa and orbital lesions can be identified through this orbital area. In contrast, the normal anatomy of the one-quarter axial view (Fig. 2b) shows the orbits and anterior portion of the middle cranial fossa obliterated by overlying activity in the facial tissues, sinuses, and middle cerebral vessels.

Some authors[7] have utilized lateral as well as anterior views in their scan procedures. Interference from radioactivity with the opposite orbit and adnexal areas tends to decrease the amount of information available from this view and may make scan interpretation more difficult.

Radionuclide arteriography[9] has been utilized in ophthalmology to delineate orbital lesions. The technique is similar to that used for scintiphotography of the central nervous system. An *en face* view is used as in the orbital scanning technique. A study of the carotid circulation as well as the detection of vascular orbital lesions can be made on a more definitive basis.

Figure 3 demonstrates a schematic appearance of the normal dynamic scan with [99m]technetium pertechnetate. The scan is performed immediately after an injected bolus of [99m]technetium pertechnetate is administered intravenously into an antecubital vein. The patient is positioned so that the head is rigidly fixed by tape or bands with the posterior skull area directly pressed against the camera face. The times stated in the figure refer to time after injection. The most important part of the study shows flow through the internal carotids within 5 seconds and the anterior and middle cerebral arterial flow within 8 seconds. Congenital and acquired malformations of the carotid system and vascular tumors can readily be appreciated during the early flow sequences. In later sequences, the integrity of the cerebral circulation can be more thoroughly examined.

Figures 4 through 7 show patients with unilateral exophthalmos and the results of their orbital scans. The patient in Fig. 4a was a 50-year-old male who had a unilateral proptosis on the left side secondary to an endocrine imbalance, and his scan is shown in Fig. 4b. The patient shown in Fig. 5 was a 55-year-old female who had an inflammatory pseudotumor on the left side causing a unilateral proptosis, and her scan is shown in Fig. 5b. The patient shown in Fig. 6a was a 50-year-old male with a mass in the superior nasal aspect of the left orbit which was excised and proved to be a dermoid tumor

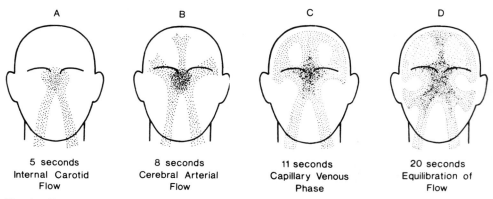

A	B	C	D
5 seconds Internal Carotid Flow	8 seconds Cerebral Arterial Flow	11 seconds Capillary Venous Phase	20 seconds Equilibration of Flow

Fig. 3. Diagrams of normal radionuclide arteriogram (A-D). Times refer to number of seconds after intravenous injection. (Courtesy of A. S. Grove, Jr. and L. M. Kotner, Jr., *Archives of Ophthalmology* 89:13–17, January 1973. Copyright 1973, American Medical Association.)

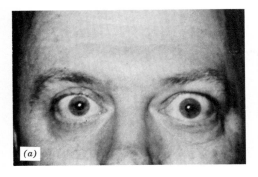
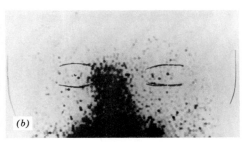

Fig. 4. (*a*) Fifty-five-year-old man with left-sided proptosis secondary to an endocrine imbalance. (*b*) Negative orbital scan of patient show in (*a*).

and the result of the negative orbital scan is shown in Fig. 6*b*. The patient shown in Fig. 7*a* was a 35-year-old female who had a neurolemmoma of the right orbit and the result of the orbital scan is shown in Fig. 7*b*.

The great majority of patients in our series with exophthalmos secondary to an endocrine imbalance had negative scans. This is similar to the series reported by Schlesinger, Trokel, and Bailey[6] using ^{197}Hg and ^{99}Tc, but differs from the series reported by Grove and Kotner[5] utilizing the same radionuclides. The two positive scans in this group of eight patients in our series were characterized only by slight increase in radionuclide localization on the affected side.

The six patients with inflammatory masses in the orbit causing the exophthalmos showed positive scans; this is similar to the two previously stated series. Most primary or secondary orbital tumors will have a positive scan. Three of nine tumor cases in our series had negative scans: one was a metastatic carcinoma from the breast, one was a malignant melanoma of the choroid with extraocular extension and the third case was a malignant lymphoma. There were two cases of benign cystic lesions of the orbit which showed negative scans, which is characteristic of cystic lesions. Cellular or vascular tumors will generally show a positive scan.

In this series of 25 cases, there were no examples of mucoceles from the paranasal

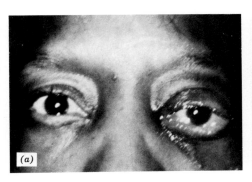
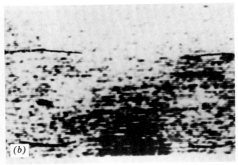

Fig. 5. (*a*) Fifty-five-year-old female with a left-side proptosis secondary to an inflammatory pseudotumor. (*b*) Scan shows diffuse increased isotope activity in left orbit.

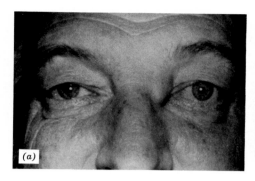 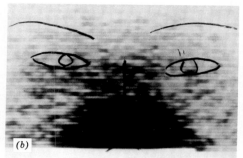

Fig. 6. (a) Fifty-year-old male with a dermoid tumor in the superior nasal aspect of the left orbit. (b) No isotope concentration in the suspected area.

sinuses; these would be expected to show negative scans. Fibrous dysplasia of the bone may show a positive scan.[7] A unilateral focal increase in radionuclide is suggestive of an orbital neoplasm or an inflammatory granuloma. A negative scan in a patient with a unilateral exophthalmos is commonly associated with endocrine dysfunction or a benign cystic lesion of the orbit.

In the three series (Flanagan and Carmichael; Schlesinger, Trokel, and Bailey, and Grove and Kotner) there were 59 orbital tumors, of which 45 demonstrated positive scans. The majority of the 14 negative scans in this group had benign cystic lesions of the orbit; however, there were 2 gliomas of the optic nerve, 1 lymphoma, and 1 metastatic breast carcinoma. In all 3 series there were 26 cases of endocrine exophthalmos, 20 of which had negative scans. Four of the positive scans in this group were from Grove and Kotner's series which showed a ring pattern of activity. This ring pattern may have been recorded because a larger dose of radionuclide had been administered or a pin point collimator was used to measure the activity response.[10] There were 16 cases of inflammatory pseudotumor of the orbit in the 3 series, 15 of which demonstrated positive scans. Vascular malformations accounted for 3 cases in the 3 series and 2 of these demonstrated positive scans.

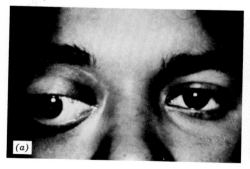 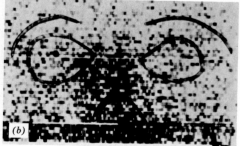

Fig. 7. (a) Thirty-five-year-old female with a neurolemmoma of the right orbit. (b) Scan shows a focal area of increased isotope concentration.

SUMMARY

Static and dynamic radionuclide scanning adds a new dimension in the diagnosis of diseases of the orbit and ocular adnexae. In any case of unilateral exophthalmos in which the diagnosis of endocrine pathology is not clear-cut, it can serve as a very useful screening tool. All patients with suspected orbital disease should have routine skull and orbital films as a complement to any scan procedure for anatomic orientation and topographic information that might be useful in delineating suspected pathology.

REFERENCES

1. Drescher, E. G. and Benedict, W. L.: Asymmetric Exophthalmos. *Arch. Ophthalmol.* **44**:109–128 (1950).

2. Reese, A. B.: *Tumors of the Eye,* 2nd ed. Harper and Row, New York, 1963, pp. 531–533.

3. Henderson, J. H.: *Orbital Tumors.* Saunders, Philadelphia, 1973, p. 26.

4. Putterman, A. M.: Evaluation of Orbital Tumors. *Ophthalmol. Dig.* **35**:34–36 (January 1973).

5. Grove, A. S., and Kotner, L. M.: Orbital Scanning with Multiple Radionuclides. *Arch. Ophthalmol.* **89**:301–305 (April 1973).

6. Schlesinger, E. B., Trokel, S. L., and Bailey, S.: Radioactive Scanning in the Analysis of Unilateral Exophthalmos. *Trans. A.A.O.O.* **73** (1969)

7. Trokel, S., Schlesinger, E. B., and Beaton H.: Diagnosis of Orbital Tumors by Gamma Ray, *Orbitography. Am. J. Ophthalmol.* **74**:675–679.

8. Wilson, E. B. and Briggs, R. C.: Study of Orbital Region Using *En Face* View. *Radiology* **92**(3):576–580 (March 1969).

9. Grove, A. S., Jr., and Kotner, L. M., Jr.: Radionuclide Arteriography in Ophthalmology. *Arch. Ophthalmol.* **89**:13–17 (1973).

10. Grove, A. S.: Personal communication. Symposium of Nuclear Medicine, Philadelphia, March 1975.

High Resolution Pinhole Scintiphotography of the Orbits and Orbital Adnexae

Robert B. Grove, M.D.
Instructor in Ophthalmology,
Harvard Medical School,
Boston, Massachusetts

Static radionuclide imaging of the orbital region has been shown by several investigators[1-8] to be of significant aid in the diagnosis and characterization of lesions involving the orbits and orbital adenexa, particularly in patients with proptosis. The procedure is rapid, without significant discomfort, and has almost no morbidity. It can help select those patients that require orbital contrast studies or, in many cases, eliminate the need for them. Various methods have been suggested for improving lesion detectability in orbital scanning, such as slight extension of the head from the usual position for anterior brain scans[5, 6] and color enhancement of the images.[4] Both the rectilinear scanner with focused collimators and the scintillation camera with nonfocusing, parallel-hole collimators have been utilized.[1, 2] All of these techniques have been hampered by the inherent lack of resolution and anatomic detail available from the imaging instrumentation employed in the study; that is, the inability to visualize lesions smaller than 1.0–1.5 cm. Reduction of this limitation would considerably enhance the clinical utility of radionuclide orbital imaging. In an effort to achieve this increase in resolution (ability to detect small lesions) and anatomic detail, the feasibility of imaging the orbits using a scintillation camera with a pinhole collimator was evaluated.

PRINCIPLE OF PINHOLE COLLIMATION

The first collimator devised for use with the gamma scintillation camera was a single pinhole aperture.[9] With the advent of newer multihole collimators, use of the pinhole has declined, but the unique advantage of magnification that it provides has been recognized, and its use has been advocated for imaging of the thyroid[10] and posterior fossa.[11]

The collimator in a scintillation detection system is analogous to the lens in a conventional-light camera system. It is the portion of the system that directs our vision toward and determines the manner in which we view a target. Through the use of different lenses (collimators), varying projections of the target can be presented to the film (scintillation crystal).

Any scintillation imaging system has a certain degree of intrinsic resolution; that is, without the collimator, it can detect lesions of a certain minimum size. If an object to be imaged contains a lesion that is smaller than this minimum detectable size, and the object is presented to the system by the collimator in a 1:1 relationship, it will not be detected. However, if the object could be magnified by the collimator so that the lesion appears greater than the minimum detectable size when it is presented to the detector, it could then be visualized.

A schematic diagram of the principle of pinhole collimation is shown in Fig. 1. As long as the distance from the pinhole aperture to the target is smaller than the distance from the pinhole aperture to the scintillation crystal, a magnified, inverted representation of the target is presented to the crystal. Since the inherent resolution of the scintillation camera system begins at the crystal, presentation of a magnified image of the target to the crystal results in an increase in effective resolution. What was a lesion initially too small to be visualized by the scintillation system can, given the necessary amount of magnification, be brought within its ability to detect. Nothing in the system has changed, except the manner in which the target is presented to the detector.

The increase in resolution that can be obtained with a pinhole collimator is directly proportional to the amount of magnification it provides. The magnification factor varies,

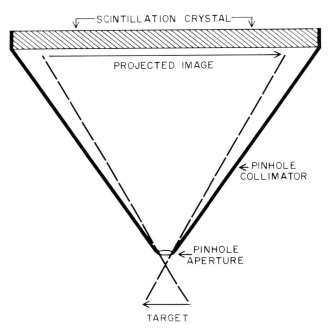

Fig. 1. Principle of pinhole collimation. Magnified, inverted image of target is projected through pinhole aperture onto scintillation crystal. Magnification occurs as long as distance from pinhole aperture to target is less than distance from pinhole aperture to crystal.

increasing as the distance from the pinhole aperture to the target decreases. The size of lesions that can be detected is limited by the size of the pinhole aperture. Lesions smaller than the pinhole diameter will not be visualized.

The image quality produced by scintillation detection systems is determined by several factors, but the most important of these are resolution and sensitivity. Within any given system, these important parameters are inversely related. Consequently, the increased resolution provided by the pinhole collimator results in decreased sensitivity (counts detected/photons emitted) of the system, and a longer time required to obtain a satisfactory information density (counts per square centimeter) in the images. This longer time required to obtain the necessary number of counts for a high-quality image is minimized by the use of high photon-yield radionuclides such as technetium.

METHOD

Patients with ophthalmological findings or a clinical history suggesting orbital or retroorbital lesions were studied. Each patient received 800 mg of potassium perchlorate orally 30 minutes prior to the administration of ^{99m}Tc-pertechnetate. Perchlorate reduces the uptake of pertechnetate by the salivary glands and thyroid. A dose of 20–25 mCi of ^{99m}Tc-pertechnetate was then given intravenously, after which a routine four-view brain scan, an *en face* (anterior orbital) view, and pinhole orbital views at various degrees of magnification were obtained. In most instances, imaging was performed between 30 and 90 minutes postinjection. Delayed views at 3 to 4 hours postinjection were obtained in selected patients. In all images 300,000 to 500,000 counts were obtained, requiring from 4 to 9 minutes with the pinhole system.

A majority of the patients were studied using a Searle Phogamma III HP camera with the standard Searle pinhole collimator having a 5 mm pinhole aperture and a pinhole-to-crystal distance of 19 cm. In several cases, the system used was an Ohio-Nuclear Series-100 camera utilizing the standard Ohio-Nuclear pinhole collimator with a 5 mm pinhole aperture and a pinhole-to-crystal distance of 23 cm. Images from the Ohio-Nuclear camera were also displayed and processed using an Ohio-Nuclear Series 150 data system.

The magnification factor of the Pho-gamma system at various pinhole-to-target distances was determined by imaging a 3 cm column of technetium in a capillary tube, first with a high resolution parallel hole collimator in contact with the target and then with the pinhole collimator beginning at 8 in. and decreasing to ½ in. As shown in Fig. 2a, a maximum magnification factor of 6.2 was obtained at ½ in. from the target.

A resolution comparison between the high-resolution, parallel-hole collimator and the pinhole was performed to estimate the size of lesions which might be detected (Fig. 2b). The target was a Picker thyroid phantom filled with technetium and containing a 6 mm cold lesion in the right upper pole. This small lesion was not detected with the parallel hole collimator, but it was easily visualized with the pinhole system. Similar quantita-

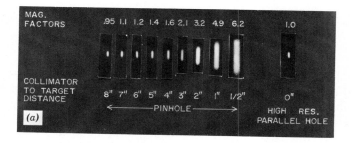

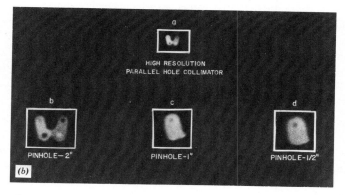

Fig. 2. (a) Magnification factors of pinhole collimator at different pinhole-to-target distances compared to high resolution (res.) parallel hole collimator in contact with target. Magnification increases as pinhole-to-target distance decreases. Maximum magnification of 6.2 at 1/2 in. from target. (b) Resolution of pinhole collimator compared to high-resolution, parallel-hole collimator. Target is technetium-filled Picker thyroid phantom having 6 mm cold lesion in right upper pole. Lesion not seen with parallel-hole collimator (a), but well-visualized with higher magnification pinhole views (c and d).

tion of the magnification factors and resolution of the Ohio-Nuclear pinhole system showed comparable results.

The standard position was used for routine anterior brain images, with the orbitomeatal line perpendicular to the parallel-hole, high-resolution collimator. Anterior orbital views were obtained with the head extended 15° from this position. The position used for pinhole orbital views is shown in Fig. 3. Initial pinhole views were obtained with the collimator centered over the bridge of the patient's nose at a point halfway between the superior and inferior orbital rims and approximately 2 in. from the globes. The orbitomeatal line is extended 15°–20° from the longitudinal axis of the collimator. This position allows maximal visualization of both orbits simultaneously. Subsequently, with the patient in this same position, the collimator can be centered over each orbit at a distance of ½ in. to obtain individual views of each orbit at maximal magnification. Because of the magnification obtained with the pinhole, accurate alignment without rotation is essential so that the resultant images are symmetrical and allow direct comparison of corresponding areas. The patients should be instructed to close their eyes and maintain the globes as still as possible throughout the study.

RESULTS

Eleven patients with various disease processes involving the orbits and orbital adenexae have been studied, and the results are summarized in Table 1. There were nine studies in which an abnormality was demonstrated, while two were considered to be normal.

Patient 1.   A 58-year-old male had a pigmented 4 × 6 mm choroidal mass in the right eye which had been stable over a 2-year period and which was not visualized. Figure 4a shows a normal pinhole orbital image at 2 in., demonstrating the symmetrical orbits outlined by a peripheral rim of activity with central clear zones in the area of the globes. Normal midline nasopharyngeal and saggital sinus activity is also seen. Figure 4b and c show the normal image of each orbit obtained with the pinhole centered over

TABLE 1. SUMMARY—PINHOLE ORBIT STUDIES

Patient No.	Diagnosis	Scan Results	
		Negative	Positive
1.	Pigmented choroidal mass, 4 × 6 mm. Stable—2 yr.	X	
2.	Malignant melanoma of choroid, 4 × 5 mm		X
3.	Sphenoid ridge meningioma		X
4.	Subretinal chronic hematoma, 5 × 6 mm		X
5.	Pseudotumor of orbit		X
6.	Pseudotumor of orbit		X
7.	Eye changes of chronic Graves' disease—Class 3		X
8.	Optic neuritis	X	
9.	Malignant melanoma of orbit		X
10.	Postop sphenoid ridge meningioma		X
11.	Von Hipple Lindau ocular angioma		X
11	Totals	2	9

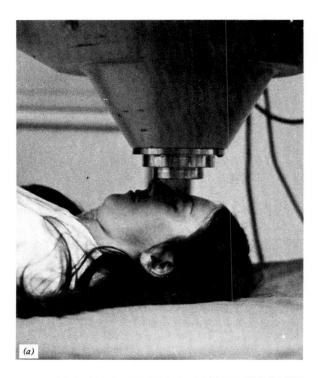

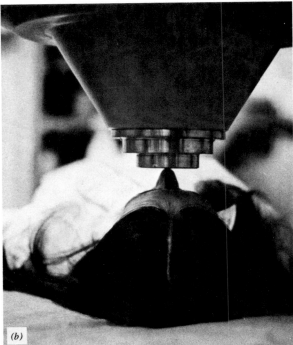

Fig. 3.   Position for initial pinhole orbital views. (a) Pinhole aperture centered over bridge of nose, halfway between superior and inferior orbital rims, at distance of 2 in. Orbitomeatal line extended 15°–20° from longitudinal axis of collimator. (b) alignment must be straight with no rotation of patient's head.

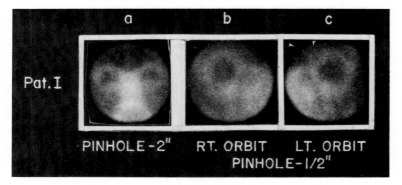

Fig. 4.   Patient 1: (a) Normal pinhole image at 2 in. encompassing both orbits. (b) and (c) Normal pinhole images of individual orbits at 1/2 in.

each globe at a distance of ½ in., providing maximum magnification and detail. With maximum magnification, the peripheral rim of uptake can be seen to include three areas of slightly increased activity located superiolaterally, superiomedially, and inferiomedially, which probably represent normal accumulation of ^{99m}Tc-pertechnetate in the lacrimal apparatus.

Patient 2.   A 34-year-old female had a 4 × 5 mm malignant melanoma of the choroid in the left eye. The size of this tumor can be appreciated in Fig. 5c. Fig. 5a shows her anterior orbital scintigram, which is normal. The pinhole orbital view (Fig. 5b) at 2 in. detected the tumor, showing a definite rounded area of increased uptake superiomedially in the clear zone of the left globe.

Patient 3.   A 42-year-old female presented with a 5-year history of progressive visual loss in the left eye with minimal proptosis and left frontal headaches. She had a superior temporal field cut on the left and anisocoria with the left pupil smaller than the right. No other focal neurological abnormalities were noted, and both examination of the fundus and skull films were normal. Her routine anterior brain scan (Fig. 6a) showed only the suggestion of a slight asymmetry at the base on the left which might have been normal. The anterior orbital view (Fig. 6b) also showed only a minor asymmetry in the

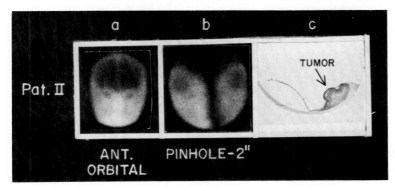

Fig. 5.   Patient 2: Malignant melanoma (4 × 5 mm) of choroid in left eye. (a) Anterior orbital view. (b) Pinhole view at 2 in. (c) Low-power photomicrograph of section of eye through tumor.

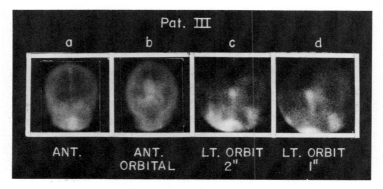

Fig. 6.   Patient 3: Meningioma of medial sphenoid ridge. (a) Anterior brain scan. (b) Anterior orbital view. (c) and (d) Pinhole views at 2 in. and 1 in., respectively.

region of the medial left orbit. However, the pinhole orbital study (Fig. 6c and d) revealed a striking asymmetry with an area of considerably increased uptake in the medial portion of the left orbit. Primarily on the basis of this study, an arteriogram was performed which demonstrated a mass lesion. At surgery, she was found to have a meningioma of the medial sphenoid ridge.

Patient 4.   A 63-year-old male had a chronic, subretinal hemorrhage, 5 × 6 mm in size, in his right eye. The anterior orbital view (Fig. 7a) was normal, and the pinhole view at 2 in. (Fig. 7b) was equivocal, but at ½ in. (Fig. 7c and d), the pinhole study demonstrated this lesion as a rounded area of increased uptake in the clear zone of the right eye.

Patient 5.   An 18-year-old male presented with pain, proptosis, and limitation of movement of the left eye. Fundus examination revealed only dilated venules without pulsations. A tumor was suspected, but a left internal and left common carotid angiogram and a left orbital venogram were normal. Subsequently, orbital scintigraphy was performed. The anterior brain scan (Fig. 8a) was equivocal, but the pinhole orbital view (Fig. 8b) revealed diffusely increased uptake of ^{99m}Tc-pertechnetate around the rim of

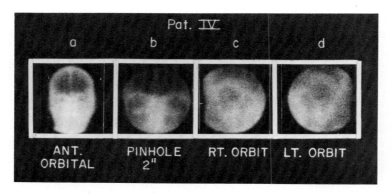

Fig. 7.   Patient 4: Chronic subretinal hemorrhage in right eye. (a) Anterior orbital view. (b) Pinhole view at 2 in. (c) and (d) Pinhole views at 1/2 in.

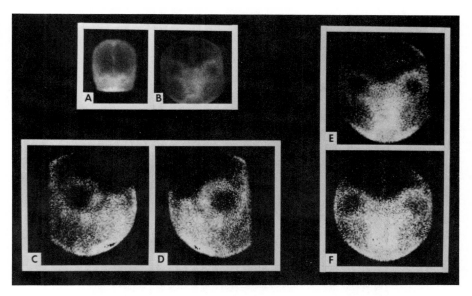

Fig. 8.   Patient 5: Diffuse pseudotumor of left orbit. (A) Anterior brain scan. (B) Pinhole view at 2 in. (C) and (D) Pinhole views at 1/2 in. taken from video display of data system.

the left orbit. When this image was viewed on the video display of the Ohio-Nuclear data system with added contrast (Fig. 8c,d, and e), the increased uptake around the rim of the left orbit was even more apparent. This lesion was felt to represent a diffuse orbital pseudotumor. After a course of steroid therapy, the asymmetry of uptake around the left orbital rim had diminished (Fig. 8f) and the proptosis resolved.

Patient 7.   A 44-year-old female developed Graves' disease with eye changes. She had been euthyroid and her eye changes stable. However, she had recently experienced eye pain, left greater than right, and slight progression of proptosis on the left. Pinhole orbital views showed the right orbit to be relatively normal (Fig. 9b and d) but revealed slightly increased uptake around the left orbital rim and diffusely increased activity in the clear zone of the left orbit (Fig. 9c and e).

Patient 10.   A 52-year-old female had surgery for a left sphenoid ridge meningioma in 1970 and again in 1972. In early 1974, she had progressive visual loss in the left eye and papilledema. She had a third craniotomy in January 1974 which revealed no evidence of recurrent tumor, but dense scarring around the left optic nerve was noted. Because of increasing seizure frequency, a brain scan and pinhole orbital study were obtained in February 1975. The anterior brain scan 30 minutes postinjection (Fig. 10a and c) and the 4-hour delayed study (Fig. 10b) showed only minor asymmetry in the left orbital region. However, pinhole orbital studies 45 minutes postinjection (Fig. 10d and f) revealed considerable abnormal uptake in and above the superiomedial left orbital rim, which was not present in the image of the right orbit (Fig. 10e). Delayed pinhole views at 4 hour postinjection (Fig. 10g and h) showed this abnormal uptake to have decreased (Fig. 10h), making it most likely that this abnormality was vascular in nature and related to her previous surgery, rather than to a recurrence of tumor in the area.

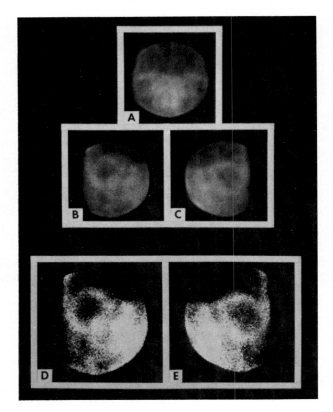

Fig. 9.   Patient 7: Eye changes of Graves disease symptomatic on left. (A) Pinhole view at 2 in. (B) and (C) Pinhole views at 1/2 in. from camera display. (D) and (E) Pinhole views from data system video display with added contrast, showing abnormality of left orbit more clearly.

DISCUSSION

The use of a pinhole collimator-gamma scintillation camera system for orbital imaging would appear to offer significant advantages over previously used scanning techniques, which, although useful, have been limited to the detection of relatively large lesions. In many of the disease processes involving the orbits and orbital adenexa, the lesions are below the detection capability of scintillation systems using parallel hole collimation. In the nine patients in this study in whom the pinhole system definitely demonstrated the lesion, routine anterior and anterior orbital brain scans were either normal or only minimally suggestive of an abnormality. The two patients with normal pinhole orbital studies both had relatively quiescent disease processes with little tissue reaction. Such lesions would not be expected to accumulate significant amounts of ^{99m}Tc-pertechnetate.

Not only does the image magnification provided by the pinhole system result in a significant increase in the ability to detect very small lesions but also greater anatomic detail is available for characterization of the abnormality. The marked increase in resolution obtained with the pinhole system compensates for its disadvantage of decreased sensitivity. Because of the physical characteristics of technetium,[13] a large dose (25 mCi)

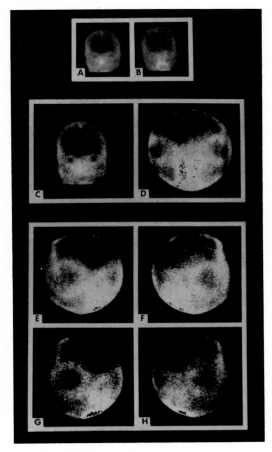

Fig. 10.   Patient 10: Left sphenoid wing meningioma removed on two occasions. Evaluation for possible recurrence. (A) and (C) Anterior orbital view 30 min. postinjection. (B) 4 hour delayed anterior orbital view. (D) 30 minute pinhole view at 2 in. (E) and (F) Pinhole views at 1/2 in. done at 30 minutes. (G) and (H) 4 hour delayed pinhole views at 1/2 in.

can be used with minimal radiation exposure to the patient (0.4 rad whole body), and the time required for imaging is not excessive.

A considerable amount of normal activity is seen in the area of the nasopharynx, which could possibly cause problems in interpretation of the orbital images, particularly if nasopharyngeal uptake is asymmetric. Administration of atropine in appropriate dosage prior to injection of the radiopharmaceutical should serve to reduce the nasopharyngeal accumulation of pertechnetate. However, in this group of patients in whom atropine was not used, nasopharyngeal activity did not hinder interpretation of the pinhole images. Due to the anatomic detail present in the pinhole studies performed at maximum magnification (Fig. 4b and c), a zone of relatively decreased activity is seen between the ring of uptake surrounding the orbital rim and the nasopharyngeal activity.

The ring of pertechnetate localization surrounding the orbits is due to the presence of the radiopharmaceutical in the normal vascularity of the orbital tissues, lacrimal apparatus, and muscles. The central clear zones are due to the relatively avascular globes. The increased pertechnetate uptake in lesions is most likely related to their abnormal vascularity and/or inflammation.

An important aspect of interpretation of the pinhole orbital images is the presence or absence of the generally symmetrical uptake which should be evident in a normal study. The initial pinhole view at a distance of 2 in. (Fig. 4a) provides the greatest degree of magnification which maintains a field of view sufficient to include both orbits in the same image. Larger lesions should be apparent as an abnormal asymmetry in this view. Careful positioning is required for the pinhole views of each individual orbit performed at ½ in. (Fig. 4b and c) so that the position of the orbital rims and the amount of periorbital structures included in each image is approximately the same, permitting the presence or absence of symmetry to be evaluated. Difficulty may be encountered in patients with a bilateral process, since the images may be symmetrically abnormal.

Questions have been raised in several studies concerning distortion produced by the pinhole collimator.[14, 15, 16] The field response of the pinhole collimator is nonuniform, but the nonuniformity is predictable.[17, 18] Figure 11 shows the field response of the Searle 5 mm pinhole collimator 2 in. from a uniform flood source of technetium. Using a Nuclear Data 50/50 med computer, the field response was vertically displayed. There was a 33% reduction in response at the edge of the field compared to the center, but the variation in response was gradual and symmetrical around the center of the field.

In addition, the rapidly divergent field of view of the pinhole collimator can cause geometric distortion unless the target is maintained parallel to the plane of the scintillation crystal. The potential problem with distortion using the pinhole collimator was of no clinical importance in the orbital images obtained in this study. As long as symmetry is maintained in the images and proper positioning with the orbits parallel to the scintillation crystal is utilized, any distortion that may be introduced will be balanced and represent an insignificant problem.

The ability to vary image contrast on a video display was useful in interpretation of the studies in several patients. Increasing contrast can in some cases make abnormalities

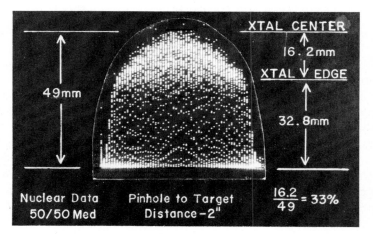

Fig. 11. Flood field response of Searle 5 mm pinhole collimator 2 in. from uniform sheet source of technetium. Response displayed vertically using Nuclear Data 50/50 Med computer. Response at edge of crystal (xtal) is 33% less than at center of crystal, but is symmetrical about the center of the field.

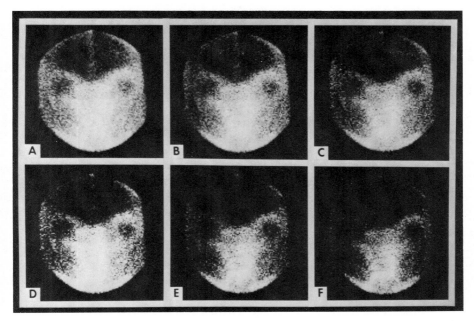

Fig. 12. Effect of increasing image contrast using data-system video display on ability to visualize lesion. Images (patient 5—pseudotumor of left orbit) have increasing contrast from zero (A) to 5 units (F).

much more apparent (Fig. 12), but must be utilized judiciously, since excessive contrast can mask subtle areas of abnormal radionuclide accumulation.

Radionuclide orbital scanning is useful in the initial diagnosis and characterization of lesions involving the orbits and in the subsequent evaluation of therapy or recurrence of disease. The procedure is simple, rapid, and without significant risk to the patient. Further investigation will be required before the full value of the pinhole technique for orbital imaging becomes apparent, but it should serve to significantly enhance the utility of nuclear medicine studies in this area.

REFERENCES

1. Grove, A. S., Jr., and Kotner, L. M., Jr.: Orbital Scanning with Multiple Radionuclides. *Arch. Ophthalmol.* **89**:301–305 (1973).
2. Schlesinger, E. B., Trokel, S. L., and Bailey, S.: Radioactive Scanning in the Analysis of Unilateral Exophthalmos. *Trans. Am. Acad. Ophthalmol. Otolaryngol.* **73**:1005–1012 (1969).
3. Trokel, S. L., Schlesinger, E. B., and Beaton, H.: Diagnosis of Orbital Tumors by Gamma-Ray Orbitography. *Am. J. Ophthalmol.* **74**:675–679 (1972).
4. Kramer, S. G. et al: Color Enhancement of Brain and Orbital Scans in Proptosis. *Trans. Am. Acad. Ophthalmol. Otolaryngol.* **74**:1240–1247 (1970).
5. Kramer, S. G., and Polcyn, R. E.: Extension of the Head for Orbital Scanning in Proptosis. *Am. J. Ophthalmol.* **69**:284–296 (1970).
6. Wilson, E. B., Briggs, R. C.: A Study of the Orbital Region in Brain Scanning Using the en Face View. *Radiology* **92**:576–580 (1969).
7. Grove, A. S., Jr., and Kotner, L. M., Jr.: Radioisotope Evaluation of Orbital Lesions. *Trans. Am. Acad. Ophthalmol. Otolaryngol.* **75**:946 (1971).

8. Di Chiro G., Ashburn W. L., and Grove A. S., Jr.: Which Radioisotopes for Brain Scanning? *Neurology* **18**:225–236 (1968).

9. Anger, H. O.: Gamma-Ray and Positron Scintillation Camera. *Nucleonics* **21**:56–59 (1963).

10. Hurley, P. J. et al: The Scintillation Camera with Pinhole Collimator in Thyroid Imaging. *Radiology* **101**:133–138 (1971).

11. Heck, L. L., and Gottschalk, A.: Use of the Pinhole Collimator for Imaging the Posterior Fossa on Brain Scans. *Radiology* **101**:443–444 (1971).

12. Dowdey J. E., and Bonte F. J.: Principles of Scintillation Camera Image Magnification with Multichannel Convergent Collimators. *Radiology* **104**:89–96 (July 1972).

13. Wagner, H. N., Jr.: *Principles of Nuclear Medicine.* Saunders, Philadelphia, 1968, pp. 664.

14. Hayes, M.: Is Field Size Enlargement with Divergent and Pinhole Collimators Acceptable? *Radiology* **95**:525–528 (1970).

15. Fink, D. W., and Wilcox, F. W.: Field Uniformity Distortion with the Pinhole Collimator on the Scintillation Camera. *J. Nucl. Med.* **13**:338–339 (1972).

16. Cradduck, T. D.: Distortion Produced by Pinhole Collimators. *J. Nucl. Med.* **13**:778–779 (1972).

17. Mallard, J. R., and Myers, M. J.: The Performance of a Gamma Camera for the Visualization of Radioactive Isotopes in Vivo. *Phys. Med. Biol.* **8**:165–182 (1963).

18. Paix, D.: Pinhole Imaging of Gamma Rays. *Phys. Med. Biol.* **12**:489–500 (1967).

Index